Fast Facts

Fast Facts:
Gynecologic Oncology

Second edition

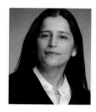

Shohreh Shahabi MD FACOG

Chair, Department of Obstetrics & Gynecology
Danbury Hospital and Chair, Reproductive Tumor Biology
Biomedical Research Laboratory, Danbury
Connecticut, USA

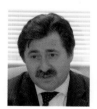

J Richard Smith MD FRCOG

Consultant Gynaecological Surgeon
West London Gynaecological Cancer Centre
Queen Charlotte's and Chelsea Hospital
Imperial College Healthcare NHS Trust, London, UK, and
Adjunct Associate Professor, New York University Medical
Center, New York, USA

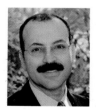

Giuseppe Del Priore MD MPH

Mary Fendrich Hulm
Director of Gynecolo
Indiana University S
Indianapolis, USA

D1464931

Declaration of Independence
This book is as balanced and as practical as we can make it.
Ideas for improvement are always welcome: feedback@fastfacts.com

HEALTH PRESS

Fast Facts: Gynecologic Oncology
First published 1998
Second edition June 2010

Book orders can be placed by telephone or via the website.
For regional distributors or to order via the website, please go to:
www.fastfacts.com
For telephone orders, please call 01752 202301 (UK), +44 1752 202301 (Europe),
1 800 247 6553 (USA, toll free), +1 419 281 1802 (Americas) or +61 (0)2 9698 7755
(Asia–Pacific).

Fast Facts is a trademark of Health Press Limited.

A CIP record for this title is available from the British Library.

ISBN 978-1-903734-00-1

Shahabi (Shohreh)
Fast Facts: Gynecologic Oncology/
Shohreh Shahabi, J Richard Smith, Giuseppe Del Priore

Acknowledgment
Chapter 9, 'Pain management and palliation' draws on chapter 6 of the previous
edition, which was written by Dr Andrew Lawson, a consultant in pain management
at the Chelsea and Westminster Hospital, London.

Medical illustrations by Dee McLean, London, UK.
Typesetting and page layout by Zed, Oxford, UK.
Printed by Latimer Trend & Company Limited, Plymouth, UK.

Text printed on biodegradable and recyclable paper
manufactured using elemental chlorine free (ECF)
wood pulp from well-managed forests.

FSC

Mixed Sources
Product group from well-managed
forests and other controlled sources

Cert no. SGS-COC-005493
www.fsc.org
© 1996 Forest Stewardship Council

Glossary of abbreviations

ACOG: American College of Obstetricians and Gynecologists

ASC-H: atypical squamous cells, cannot exclude high-grade cytology

ASC-US: atypical squamous cells of undetermined significance

BMI: body mass index

BSO: bilateral salpingo-oophorectomy

CA125: cancer antigen 125

CA19-9: cancer antigen 19-9

CIN: cervical intraepithelial neoplasia

CT: computed tomography

D&C: dilatation and curettage

EBRT: external beam radiotherapy

FDA: Food and Drug Administration

FIGO: International Federation of Gynecology and Obstetrics

GTN: gestational trophoblastic neoplasia

hCG: human chorionic gonadotropin

HIV: human immunodeficiency virus

HNPCC: hereditary non-polyposis colorectal cancer

HPV: human papillomavirus

HSIL: high-grade squamous intraepithelial lesion

HSV: herpes simplex virus

5HT$_3$: type three 5-hydroxytryptamine

IMRT: intensity-modulated radiotherapy

LDH: lactate dehydrogenase

LEEP: loop electrosurgical excision procedure

LLETZ: large loop excision of the transformation zone

LSIL: low-grade squamous intraepithelial lesion

LVSI: lymph–vascular space invasion

MRI: magnetic resonance imaging

NSAID: non-steroidal anti-inflammatory drug

Pap smear: Papanicolaou smear

PCA: patient-controlled analgesia

PCOS: polycystic ovary syndrome

PET: positron emission tomography

SIL: squamous intraepithelial lesion

STD: sexually transmitted disease

TNM: tumor–node–metastasis

TVUS: transvaginal ultrasound

VAIN: vaginal intraepithelial neoplasia

VIN: vulvar intraepithelial neoplasia

VLP: virus-like particle

WHO: World Health Organization

Introduction

Gynecologic oncology is a well-established subspecialty of gynecology. However, management of gynecologic malignancy is still often shared between the general gynecologist, gynecologic oncologist, radiation oncologist, medical oncologist, primary care provider and, occasionally, the palliative care specialist. Women, too, are requesting information as they become increasingly aware of their risk of genital tract malignancy, particularly as a result of the cervical screening program, the increasing publicity given to attempts to develop screening tests for ovarian cancer, and the increased risk of endometrial cancer among an aging and more obese population.

To put the burden of gynecologic cancers into perspective, the estimated numbers of new cases and deaths in the USA in 2009 are shown in Table 1.

The incidence of cervical cancer is declining in industrialized countries, almost certainly because of the implementation of cervical smear programs. It remains true, however, that those women most in need of screening or human papillomavirus vaccines are those least likely to be included in such programs. There is still much room for

TABLE 1

Estimated new cases of, and deaths from, gynecologic cancers in the USA in 2009

Site	New cases	Deaths
Uterus	42 160	7780
Ovary	21 550	14 600
Cervix	11 270	4070
Vulva	3580	900
Vagina and other	2160	770

Data from Jemal A, Siegel R, Ward E et al. Cancer statistics, 2009. *CA Cancer J Clin* 2009;59:225–49.

improvement as the projected number of new cervical cancers worldwide is anticipated to reach 2 million by 2020.

At present, 21 000 new cases of ovarian cancer are diagnosed each year in the USA, and over 14000 deaths occur annually. Worldwide, it is a leading cause of cancer deaths in women. This disease accounts for 4% of all tumors in women. Unfortunately, many women present to primary care providers early in their disease with vague, non-specific complaints, making it easy to miss the underlying diagnosis. This may represent an opportunity for well-informed clinicians to intervene in a meaningful manner.

Gynecologic tumors that have a low incidence are seen infrequently by the non-subspecialist, but nevertheless they require prompt recognition and management to minimize their potentially devastating effects.

Fast Facts: Gynecologic Oncology aims to update the primary care provider and non-specialist who see these tumors infrequently on current management and prognosis. It also provides a useful starting point for medical students and junior doctors on a gynecologic oncology rotation.

The cervix

The area of the cervix with premalignant potential is the
transformation zone, which is formed after puberty. Before puberty,
the squamocolumnar junction is found inside the endocervical canal
(Figure 1.1a). At puberty, cervical eversion occurs under the influence
of estrogens, resulting in cervical ectopy (Figure 1.1b). The vagina
is then colonized by lactobacilli and the acidity increases. This
encourages squamous cell metaplasia, covering the area of cervical
ectopy (columnar epithelium) with squamous epithelium (Figure 1.1c).
Thus, there are two squamocolumnar junctions: the original one and the
new one (Figure 1.1d). The area between these is the transformation
zone, and it is this area that has the greatest premalignant potential.
This is also the area examined cytologically. Cervical ectopy is a
physiological state stimulated by increased estrogen levels; it can occur

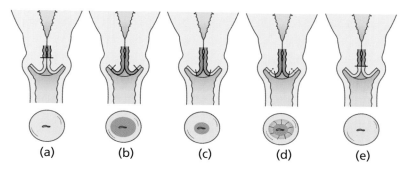

(a)   (b)   (c)   (d)   (e)

Figure 1.1 The physiological states of the cervix according to age:
(a) before puberty, the squamocolumnar junction is inside the endocervical
canal; (b) at puberty, cervical eversion occurs; (c) following puberty, the area
of cervical ectopy becomes covered with squamous epithelium; (d) two
squamocolumnar junctions result (distal older, proximal newer), and the
area between them is the transformation zone; (e) after the menopause,
the squamocolumnar junction formed following puberty ascends into the
cervical canal.

at puberty as described previously, but also occurs in women taking the combined oral contraceptive pill and during pregnancy. After the menopause, the new squamocolumnar junction ascends into the cervical canal (Figure 1.1e).

Epidemiology

Incidence. Cervical cancer has a bimodal onset in the third and sixth decades of life. The incidence of cervical cancer in the general population is uncertain, but it probably affects 8–10 women/100 000/year. However, global incidence and mortality rates are disparate. In developed countries, the incidence and mortality figures for cervical cancer have fallen by 75% over the past 50 years. In the USA from 1995 to 1999, the incidence of cervical cancer in girls aged under 20 years was 0/100 000/year, rising to 1.7/100 000/year in women aged 20–24 years, and peaking at 16.5/100 000/year in women aged 45–49 years. Only 10% of affected women were 75 or older. UK data show a similar distribution.

Approximately 60% of women who are newly diagnosed with cervical cancer in developed countries have either never been screened or not been screened in the preceding 5 years. Cervical cancer is more common in metropolitan areas than in rural areas, and the incidence is higher in populations with lower socioeconomic status and low levels of education. Central and South America, southern and eastern Africa, and the Caribbean have the highest incidence of the disease.

Risk factors. Cervical cancer is a disease associated with chronic infection by oncogenic types of human papillomavirus (HPV). The most important cofactors that affect the persistence and progression of HPV infection are HPV type and viral load. Other cofactors that may influence the outcome of HPV infection include diet, unidentified genetic factors and, possibly, other sexually transmitted disease. Host factors that influence infection include cellular and humoral immunity, parity, multiple sexual partners, smoking, pregnancy and use of oral contraceptive.

Diet. Folate deficiency is reported to enhance the effects of other risk factors such as parity, infection with type 16 HPV and cigarette smoking on the development of cervical intraepithelial neoplasia (CIN). The role of folate as a protective factor has not yet been demonstrated. In many studies, intake of other nutrients, especially vitamin C, appeared to protect against cervical cancer. Unfortunately, when administered as part of a randomized controlled trial, high-dose folic acid, vitamin C and beta-carotene supplements actually worsened CIN.

Exogenous hormones. An association between exogenous hormones and cervical disease could be explained by a number of mechanisms. For example, estrogens and progestins could directly promote permissive replication of HPV. They may also act indirectly – a reduction in blood folate levels is occasionally observed in women taking oral contraceptives, for example. Hormones produce an eversion of the columnar epithelium thus activating the HPV vulnerable, immature, squamous metaplasia.

The relative risks of cervical cancer among women using oral contraceptives for less than 5 years, 5–9 years and 10 or more years are 1.1, 1.6 and 2.2, respectively. Adenocarcinoma appears to have a stronger association with the use of oral contraceptives than squamous cell cancer. In a population regularly screened, the association is not of enough clinical significance to alter contraception recommendations, however.

Smoking. Epidemiological observations implicate smoking in this disease, and laboratory evidence suggests its role may be mediated via effects on Langerhans cells, which act as antigen-presenting cells in the local immune response in the cervix. Smoking appears to reduce the number of Langerhans cells, resulting in a decreased level of local immunity to HPV. In addition, DNA adducts (abnormal pieces of DNA covalently bonded to carcinogenic chemicals) are significantly more common in the cervical epithelium of smokers than in non-smokers, and it has been suggested that the secretion of byproducts of cigarette smoke has a mutagenic effect on the cervical epithelium. The relative risks of CIN 2 or 3 with smoking alone, HPV infection alone, and both smoking and HPV infection are approximately 2, 15 and 66, respectively, compared with HPV-negative non-smokers. The relative risk of cervical cancer is increased two- to four-fold among cigarette smokers compared with non-smokers.

Generalized immunosuppression, either iatrogenic (e.g. after renal transplantation) or as a result of immunosuppression from any cause, is associated with cervical cancer and its precursors. Women infected with human immunodeficiency virus (HIV) are often also infected with HPV, and have higher rates of cervical dysplasia and progression to invasive carcinoma than HIV-negative women. The risks of HPV infection and cervical neoplasia increase with increasing degrees of immunosuppression. The standardized incidence ratio for cervical cancer is 9.2 times higher for HIV-infected women than for women not infected with HIV. Invasive cervical cancer was designated in 1993 as an AIDS-case-defining illness by the US Centers for Disease Control and Prevention.

'Male factor'. There may be a 'male factor' involved over and above the transmission of HPV; some men have been shown to have had a number of partners who developed CIN, and semen appears to have a number of local immunosuppressive qualities. Circumcised males have a lower risk of penile HPV infection and, in those with a history of multiple partners, a reduced risk of cervical cancer in their current partners. An international study concluded that circumcision can be considered an important cofactor in the natural history of HPV infection, as it may influence the risk of HPV acquisition and transmission as well as effects on the risk of CIN. The authors recommended that, given the worldwide effect of these diseases on public health, further study is needed to determine how routine circumcision can be implemented to reduce the risks of HIV and HPV infection.

Etiology

Cervical squamous carcinoma and its precursors are largely caused by HPV infection, though cofactors may also be required, giving a multifactorial etiology. There is now considerable evidence that *Chlamydia trachomatis* and herpes simplex virus (HSV) are surrogate markers of exposure to HPV, rather than causal factors. Host immunity may be modified by these infections, thereby facilitating persistence of oncogenic HPV virus.

Human papillomavirus. Papillomaviruses are members of the A genus of the family Papovaviridae, which also includes the polyomaviruses and SV40 virus. In humans, more than 100 types of papillomavirus have been characterized. Certain types are considered high risk for the development of cervical cancer (Table 1.1).

HPV infects epithelial cells of the skin and mucous membranes, often producing local epithelial proliferation. Once the epithelium is infected, the virus can either persist in the cytoplasm or integrate with the host genome (see page 12). HPV is highly species-specific, and HPV types have significant specificity with regard to the anatomic location of the epithelium.

Infection rates. The cumulative 3-year incidence of new HPV infection is reported to be 43%, but over 90% of HPV-infected women have spontaneous resolution of the infection within 2 years, and fewer than 5% have cytologically detected CIN. The approximate rate of persistence at 6, 12 and 24 months is reported to be 50%, 33% and 10–20%, respectively. The risk of persistence is related to age; 20% of high-risk HPV infections persist in women under 25 years of age compared with a 50% rate of persistence in women over 55. Women with otherwise normal Papanicolaou (Pap) smears who have persistent HPV infection have a higher likelihood of developing invasive cervical cancer than women with normal smears and no evidence of HPV infection.

Prevalence in women with CIN or invasive cancer. HPV is found in 70–78% of women with pathologically confirmed CIN 1 and in 83–89% of women with CIN 2 or 3. The prevalence of HPV DNA in

TABLE 1.1

Genital human papillomavirus subtypes by malignant potential*

Risk	Type
Low	6, 11, 40, 42, 43, 44, 54, 61, 70, 72, 81, CP6108
Probably high	26, 53, 66
High	16, 18, 31, 33, 35, 39, 45, 51, 52, 56, 58, 59, 68, 73, 82

*Adapted from Munoz et al. *N Engl J Med* 2003;348:518.

invasive cancer is even higher; over 90% of women with squamous cell carcinomas and adenocarcinoma/adenosquamous carcinomas are HPV-positive, compared with only 16% of controls (age-matched women without cancer).

HPV types 16, 18, 35, 45 or 59 are present in 96% of adenocarcinomas. It seems that HPV 18 is more prevalent than HPV 16 in adenocarcinomas. HPV types 16, 18, 31, 35 or 45 are present in 88% of squamous cancers. HPV types 6 and 11 have been detected in only 21% of CIN 1. HPV 16 is identified in 45% of all CIN 2 and 3 lesions and HPV 18 in 7%. HPV type 6 is the most common HPV type found in association with exophytic condylomas of the male and female anogenital tract (genital warts) in adults.

Viral integration. In low-grade dysplasia, HPV is in an episomal, non-integrated state. In contrast, the virus is integrated into the human genome in more than 80% of cancers. Viral integration results in the disruption of the E1 and E2 open-reading frames and, therefore, in the loss of the transcriptional regulation of E6 and E7, with resultant overexpression of these oncoproteins. The HPV E6 protein binds to p53 and induces the cellular degradation of p53, while E7 interacts with the retinoblastoma protein (Rb), which leads to dissociation of the transcription factor E2F and promotion of cell cycle progression. The inactivated tumor suppressor genes *p53* and *Rb* are thought to be central to the host-cell transformation induced by HPV and immortalization of infected cell lines. The presence of extracellular E7 also activates cervical endothelial cells and overproduction of interleukins 6 and 8, two cytokines that are associated with progression of cervical cancer.

Progression and regression

CIN is the precursor of invasive cervical neoplasia. The CIN grades are based on histology as opposed to the squamous intraepithelial lesion (SIL) designations, which are based on cytology.

The natural history of cervical dysplasia was evaluated in a large historical cohort study of 17 000 women with an abnormal Pap smear from Toronto, Canada. The risk of progression from mild dysplasia to severe or worse dysplasia was only 1% per year, but the risk of progression from moderate dysplasia was 16% within 2 years and 25% within 5 years. The authors concluded that most of the excess risk of cervical cancer from moderate and severe dysplasias occurred within 2 years of the initial dysplastic smear.

The American Society for Colposcopy and Cervical Pathology consensus guidelines for expectant management (watchful waiting) of women with biopsy-confirmed CIN 1 and satisfactory colposcopy recommended that, after two negative smears at 6 and 12 months or a negative HPV DNA test, annual screening may be resumed. In women with access to health care, theoretically far fewer cases should ever progress from CIN to cancer.

Screening

In general terms, the purpose of a screening program is to reduce the incidence of a specific cancer within a population. However, a number of conditions must exist in order to allow a screening program to be implemented. Cervical carcinoma is the only gynecologic malignancy that currently meets the criteria for screening.

In 1952, Papanicolaou and Traut described a cervical smear technique capable of detecting abnormal cervical cytology suggestive of cervical dysplasia. The use of colposcopy as an investigative technique was originally described by Hinsellman in 1926, but it was not adopted as the investigation of choice for women with abnormal cervical cytology until the 1970s. Since then, the concept of local minimally invasive treatment has gained universal acceptance, and a 98% cure rate is possible.

Intervals. Cervical cancer has been shown to be preventable, providing the design of the screening program is appropriate. It has, however, been shown that increasing the frequency of screening beyond a certain limit gives diminishing returns (Table 1.2), particularly in cost-benefit terms. Many organizations often update their specific recommendations regarding a screening interval (e.g. in the USA, American Society for Colposcopy and Cervical Pathology, American College of Obstetricians and Gynecologists [ACOG]). However, in general, yearly screening soon after possible HPV exposure is a reasonable starting point for

TABLE 1.2

Detection rates for cervical screening at different screening intervals*

Screening interval	Proportion of cases detected
10 years	64%
5 years (UK)	84%
3 years (UK)	89%
1 year (USA)	93%

*Sexually active women are screened between the ages of 20 (or within 3 years of initiating intercourse) and 69 years.

detecting any abnormality. However, most abnormal findings will be transient and clinically insignificant. The recent focus on limiting treatments in young women may indicate screening can be delayed until the age of 30 with no consequences. In addition, if the prevention of frank cancer is the goal, testing less frequently may help to achieve this while minimizing the number of women experiencing side effects from treatment.

Individual risk assessment can then guide future decisions regarding screening intervals and method. For instance, an older woman with no risk factors and no new HPV exposure may safely omit screening after multiple normal results.

It is important to note that cervical cancer is associated with low socioeconomic class; the incidence is higher in precisely those women with least access to health care. It is important that strenuous effort is made to access the whole population when implementing a recommended screening program.

Cytological sampling

Conventional Pap smears or liquid-based methods, such as ThinPrep® (Cytyc Corporation) or SurePath™ (BD Diagnostics – Tripath), are typically used for cervical cytology. Liquid-based specimen collection facilitates currently available and anticipated ancillary tests, such as those for HPV and other sexually transmitted diseases (STDs). A method can be chosen based on factors such as the woman's age, risk factors, and tolerance for false-negative (higher with conventional Pap) versus false-positive tests (higher with liquid-based cytology). The cost and desired screening interval (combined testing is performed every 3 years, liquid-based screening and the conventional Pap are done more frequently) are important factors. The ability of the conventional Pap and liquid-based cytology to detect pre-invasive lesions is reported to be similar. The sensitivity and specificity of the conventional Pap smear are 30–87% and 70–100%, respectively, for the detection of cervical cancer and its precursors (CIN 1–3).

Systematic reviews of studies comparing conventional and liquid-based cytology have not consistently shown that liquid-based cytology detects the precursors of significant cancer more effectively than conventional cytology.

Conventional Pap smears must be taken with a spatula, with or without an endocervical brush, according to the type of cervix (Figure 1.2). The spatula should make good contact with the transformation zone. If a single device does not accommodate the anatomy of the woman's cervix, two separate devices must be used.

Once taken, the sample should be promptly applied to the glass slide using a side-to-side motion and fixed with alcohol to prevent air drying. The slide should be accurately pre-labeled, and sent to the laboratory in a shatterproof box. When followed diligently, these simple steps produce substantial improvement in the accuracy of the test. Considerable effort has been devoted to improving laboratory testing procedures, particularly using computerized screening methods to support laboratory personnel. This has been technically possible for years, but the economics of computerized screening methods have prevented their widespread use.

Poor technique. In the USA, federal law requires that laboratories re-screen 10% of randomly selected cytology smears that were originally interpreted as negative, for the purposes of quality assurance. In the past, approximately half the errors in reported results were due to laboratory mistakes, and half occurred as a result of obtaining the smear test. However, much stricter quality control in the laboratory

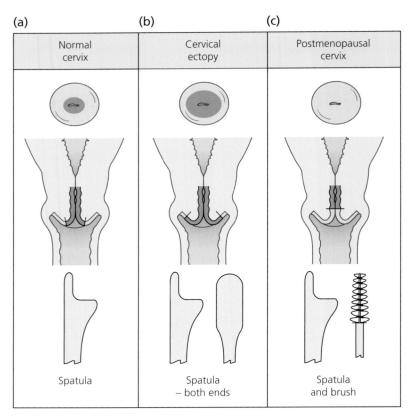

Figure 1.2 Appropriate use of spatula and brush in cervical smear testing: (a) normal cervix; (b) cervical ectopy; (c) postmenopausal cervix.

means that most false-negative results are now down to sample collection.

Liquid-based methods involve placing the cells collected into a vial of preserving liquid. The ThinPrep system involves collecting samples from the cervix in a similar manner to that used in the Pap smear except that plastic extended-tip spatulas are recommended. After the combined ectocervical and endocervical sample is obtained, the spatula is swirled vigorously in the alcohol-based preservative solution and then discarded. If a separate endocervical brush is used to obtain an endocervical sample, the brush is fully inserted into the endocervical canal and rotated a quarter or half turn in one direction. The brush is then quickly placed in the preservative solution to prevent drying and then rinsed in the solution by rotating the brush in the solution ten times while pushing against the vial wall (Figure 1.3). The brush is also swirled vigorously in the solution to release any remaining material and then the brush is discarded (not into the vial).

A proprietary broom-like device can also be used to sample the area. This device is pushed gently into the endocervical canal until it is deep enough for the shorter bristles to contact the ectocervix. It is then rotated five times in one direction to obtain the sample. The broom is removed and then pushed ten times into the bottom of a vial containing the preservative solution to force the bristles to spread apart and release the sample. Finally, the broom is swirled vigorously to further release material into the preservative solution and then the broom is discarded. A special broom-type sampling device is also used in the SurePath system. The only difference is that the entire sample is then transferred by placing the thumb against the back of the brush pad, and disconnecting the entire brush from its stem into the preservative vial.

(a)   (b)

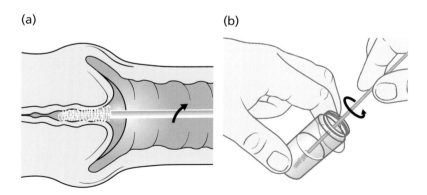

Figure 1.3 Endocervical brush for liquid-based cytology. (a) A sample is obtained from the endocervix using the endocervical brush device, which is inserted into the cervix. The device is slowly rotated for one-quarter or one-half turn in one direction. (b) The brush is rinsed quickly in the preserving liquid, pushing against the vial wall.

Direct visual inspection

Direct visual inspection with acetic acid and visual inspection with Lugol's iodine can be employed in low-resource settings as an alternative method of cervical cancer screening. Cerviscopy, speculoscopy and cervicography are different means of visually inspecting the cervix, and each provides a reasonable alternative to the typical screening regimen. In the presence of normal cytology results, a visible lesion on the cervix that is raised, friable, or has the appearance of condyloma should be biopsied regardless of the smear diagnosis. Conversely, the sensitivity of colposcopy is not as good as was once believed. A decade ago, and still for many current practitioners, colposcopy was considered the 'gold standard'. However, prospective investigations have revealed the limitation of colposcopic impression and single-directed biopsies.

HPV testing

The major indication for HPV testing in screening for cervical cancer is for triaging women with cervical cytology smears interpreted as atypical squamous cells of undetermined significance (ASC-US). HPV infection is often transient and most women with HPV infection do not develop premalignant lesions.

In the USA, the Food and Drug Administration (FDA) approved a combined test for HPV plus cervical cytology for primary screening in 2003. It is reasonable to perform combined cytology and HPV DNA testing for low-risk women aged 30 and over, and it should not be necessary more frequently than every 3 years if normal. If annual cervical screening is combined with other preventive medicine interventions, such as assessing weight or tobacco use, then annual screening may be an opportunity to intervene productively. HPV testing has also been proposed as an alternative to conventional cytology for primary screening for cervical cancer. It is reported that a negative HPV test may allow safe widening of the screening interval to 5 years.

Next steps

Cervical smear interpretation has changed over the years and the original Papanicolaou classification has been simplified. In strict scientific terms, cytology should be reported in terms of dyskaryosis or an intraepithelial lesion (Table 1.3). However, in an attempt to reduce confusion, laboratories report smear results as shown in Table 1.4. The diagnosis of CIN is only possible with histological confirmation, hence the emphasis on 'suggestive of' on cytology reports.

Atypical squamous cells are common; in fact, ASC-US is the most common abnormal result reported by most laboratories. The condition usually resolves spontaneously and is self-limited. Most actually represent a false-positive or subclinical disease. The preferred approach to ASC-US is HPV testing, with triage of women with high-risk HPV types detected to colposcopy (Table 1.5). ASC-US is most often associated with no other manifestation or sign of disease on colposcopic impression or biopsy histology. The risk of invasive cancer in women with atypical squamous cells is low (0.1–0.2%).

Suspected high-grade dysplasia. Some type of further investigation is necessary if underlying high-grade dysplasia is suspected with ASC cytology (i.e. if the woman has 'atypical squamous cells, cannot exclude

TABLE 1.3

Classification of cervical cytology

ASC-US	Atypical squamous cells of undetermined significance
ASC-H	Atypical squamous cells, cannot exclude HSIL
LSIL	Low-grade squamous intraepithelial lesion
	Encompasses:
	• HPV-related changes
	• mild dysplasia
	• mild cervical intraepithelial neoplasia (CIN)
HSIL	High-grade squamous intraepithelial lesion
	Encompasses:
	• moderate and severe dysplasia
	• moderate and severe CIN
	• carcinoma in situ

TABLE 1.4

UK and US* system for reporting results from cervical smears

Result	Action
Normal	Repeat as per national policy
Inflammatory/borderline	Screen for STDs Repeat at 6 months
Suggestive of HPV, LSIL, atypia Borderline/CIN 1	Options include colposcopy, repeat smear in 6 months or HPV testing
Suggestive of HSIL CIN 2 and 3	Colposcopy

*The latest detailed updates are available from the American Society for Colposcopy and Cervical Pathology website (www.asccp.org).
CIN, cervical intraepithelial neoplasia; HPV, human papillomavirus; HSIL, high-grade squamous intraepithelial lesion; LSIL, low-grade squamous intraepithelial lesion; STD, sexually transmitted disease.

high-grade cytology' [ASC-H]), as 24–94% of women with ASC-H have precancerous lesions (CIN 2 or 3) at biopsy compared with 5–17% of women with ASC. If an ASC-H result is reported, the woman should be referred for colposcopy, regardless of HPV testing. Over 70% of women under 30 with ASC-H test positive for HPV; the prevalence of HPV is much lower in women aged 30 or older. Therefore, HPV testing can be considered for triaging to colposcopy in older women (Table 1.5). A negative HPV test has an excellent negative predictive value.

Adolescent girls are not routinely screened in the UK, but in the USA they may have serial cytology at 6 and 12 months as HPV is highly transient; HPV DNA testing at 12 months may also be considered, with referral to colposcopy for those with positive results (atypical squamous cells or higher-grade cytology, high-risk HPV DNA types and ASC-US plus HPV-positive).

Pregnant women with ASC-US are managed in the same way as those who are not pregnant, though endocervical sampling is often avoided. The endocervical canal can be safely sampled during

TABLE 1.5

Management of women with results from HPV DNA testing and cervical cytology

Results of cytology/ HPV DNA detection*	Recommended follow-up
Negative/negative	Routine screening in 3 years
Negative/positive	Repeat combined test in 6–12 months[†]
ASC-US/negative	Repeat cytology in 12 months[‡]
ASC-US/positive	Colposcopy
Greater than ASC-US/positive or negative	Colposcopy

*Positive, high-risk HPV types are present; negative, high-risk HPV types are not present.
[†]If negative/negative, resume screening in 3 years; if ASC-US/negative, repeat combined test in 12 months; if greater than ASC-US/negative, then proceed to colposcopy; if any cytology result/positive, proceed to colposcopy.
[‡]Follow-up depends on cytology results.
ASC-US, atypical squamous cells of undetermined significance; HPV, human papillomavirus.
Adapted from Wright et al. 2004.

pregnancy using a cytobrush if clinically indicated, but the woman should be warned of the risk of bleeding.

HIV-infected women with ASC-US can be referred for immediate colposcopy rather than HPV testing or serial cytology.

Infection. The presence of bacterial vaginal infection requires treatment and then further evaluation of ASC-US. After treatment, women with high-risk HPV types are referred for colposcopy.

Cervical intraepithelial abnormalities. Treatment, when indicated, is mostly done after a histological abnormality is found on tissue biopsy directed by colposcopic impression. Cytological diagnosis alone is never enough for treatment. However, a significantly abnormal cytology result in combination with an abnormal colposcopic examination can sometimes justify immediate treatment at the time of the initial colposcopy/biopsy in women judged to be at high risk of loss to follow-up.

Pregnant, adolescent and HIV-negative women. Expectant management of these women with biopsy-confirmed CIN 1 is the preferred alternative to ablative/excisional therapy. Observation of CIN 2 or 3 for 6 to 12 months may also be appropriate in these groups.

HIV-infected women using effective antiviral medications with low viral loads and stable CD4 levels can be managed as non-HIV-infected women. Ablation and excision are both acceptable for HIV-infected women with satisfactory colposcopic examinations and biopsy-proven persistent CIN.

Colposcopy

Colposcopy is a diagnostic technique used for microscopic examination of the lower genital tract, including the cervix, vagina, anus and vulva. The organs are viewed under magnifications of between four and 20 times normal. There are no absolute contraindications to colposcopy, but acute cervicitis and vulvovaginitis should be evaluated and treated before colposcopy if possible. Postmenopausal women with an atrophic cervix may benefit from a 3-week course of topical or oral estrogen before the procedure.

Before the colposcopy is performed, an abbreviated gynecologic history is taken and an explanation given to each patient. This should cover the following points:

- smears are designed to detect precancer not cancer
- the woman's doctor thought her cervix looked normal (assuming he or she did) and cancer is unlikely
- CIN and its potential for malignant change evolves over a long period of time only if untreated
- the available treatments
- the unlikely option of 'see and treat' or, more commonly, 'wait for punch biopsy confirmation' before treatment.

The woman is placed in the lithotomy position and examined colposcopically. The exact method depends on the individual colposcopist but, in general, the procedure starts with a repetition of the cervical cytology under colposcopic guidance. Repeat cytology is actually unnecessary unless there has been a long delay since the referring result was obtained. Cytology is followed by the application of acetic acid (3% or 5%). The colposcopist then looks for areas of acetowhite (indicative of abnormal squamous lesions), taking a biopsy from any areas identified. The sensitivity of colposcopic-directed biopsies can be improved by taking more than one biopsy. The results of the colposcopy determine the next course of action.

Treatment of cervical abnormality

Figure 1.4 shows the various treatment options following colposcopy. Ablative procedures and excisional procedures are the two common

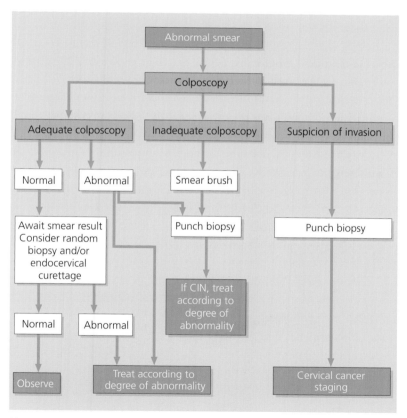

Figure 1.4 Treatment options following an abnormal smear (abnormal = CIN 2, CIN 3 or persistent CIN 1). Algorithms to aid practice in the USA are available from the American Society for Colposcopy and Cervical Pathology website (www.asccp.org). CIN, cervical intraepithelial neoplasia.

approaches. CIN 1 can be treated, but this is not a usual recommendation unless it is persistent. Severe cervical dysplasia (CIN 2 and CIN 3) requires the entire affected area of the transformation zone to be removed (Figure 1.5). No significant differences have been found between treatment modalities for CIN 2 and CIN 3 in terms of outcome (Table 1.6).

Some women are excessively anxious about pelvic examination, and this makes them unsuitable for outpatient treatment. Occasionally, such anxiety precludes outpatient examination. These women should be investigated and treated, with sedation or, more rarely, under general anesthesia.

Ablative treatment procedures remove the abnormal tissue; they do not produce a specimen for additional histological evaluation. Ablative treatment techniques include cryotherapy and laser ablation.

Ablative procedures can be performed if the following criteria are met:
- accurate histological diagnosis
- no discrepancy between cytology/colposcopy/histology

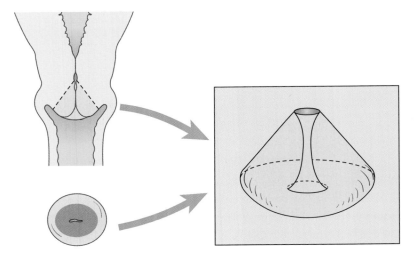

Figure 1.5 Local treatment of the transformation zone.

TABLE 1.6

Treatments for CIN 2 and 3

Treatment	Efficacy	Anesthesia	Tissue sample
Cryotherapy	> 90%	None/local	No
Laser ablation	95–98%	Local	No
Needle point electrodiathermy cone biopsy	95–98%	General	Yes
Laser conization	95–98%	Local	Yes
LLETZ/LEEP	95–98%	Local	Yes

CIN, cervical intraepithelial neoplasia; LEEP, loop electrosurgical excision procedure; LLETZ, large loop excision of the transformation zone.

- no evidence of microinvasion/invasion
- no evidence of a glandular lesion with a satisfactory colposcopy
- no evidence of endocervical involvement.

Cryotherapy refers to the application of a supercooled probe (liquid nitrous oxide or carbon dioxide) directly to the cervical lesion using one or more cooling and thawing cycles. The probe must be able to cover the entire lesion and the lesion cannot extend into the endocervical canal. Anesthesia is not required. Other advantages include ease of use, low cost and a low complication rate. The disadvantages are copious vaginal discharge lasting for weeks, a lack of tissue for histology and the use of a probe which is not easily adjusted to the dimensions of the lesion and cervix. The success rate is apparently lower than the rates associated with other methods, and cryotherapy is therefore used only for CIN 1/ low-grade squamous intraepithelial lesion (LSIL) by some practitioners.

Carbon dioxide laser ablation is both precise and flexible. Tissue is vaporized to a depth of at least 7 mm to ensure the bases of the deepest glands are destroyed. The procedure is associated with mild cramps and post-treatment vaginal discharge lasting 1–2 weeks. The technique is expensive, requires significant training and attention to safety issues, and the tissue destruction precludes detection of occult invasion through histological evaluation.

Excisional procedures excise the area of abnormality and allow further histological study. Excisional treatment can be performed by cold-knife conization, laser conization, or the loop electrosurgical excision procedure (LEEP), also called large loop excision of the transformation zone (LLETZ).

Excisional treatments should be used in the following situations

- suspected microinvasion
- unsatisfactory colposcopy (the transformation zone is not fully visualized)
- lesion involves endocervical canal
- endocervical dysplasia
- discrepancy between the cytology and colposcopy/biopsies
- suspected adenocarcinoma in situ
- invasive disease cannot be excluded
- recurrence after an ablative procedure.

Cold-knife cone biopsy (removing the transformation zone to a depth of 2.5 cm) was historically both the diagnostic tool and the treatment of choice for cervical abnormality, before outpatient treatments became available. The procedure provides a specimen without thermal marginal artifacts, so histological assessments are accurate. This is particularly important for lesions extending into the endocervical canal, suspected adenocarcinoma in situ and suspected microinvasion. Cold-knife conization appears to be associated with a lower incidence of positive margins and recurrent disease when used for the diagnosis and treatment of adenocarcinoma in situ compared with LEEP. The procedure requires general anesthesia, and the major disadvantage is that some women subsequently develop cervical incompetence or stenosis. A fine tip 'needle' cautery has been shown, in a randomized trial, to be superior to cold-knife conization performed with a scalpel, as the needle tip is more hemostatic.

LEEP (or LLETZ) has become the approach of choice for treating CIN 2 and 3 because of its ease of use, low cost and high rate of success. It can be performed readily in the clinic using local anesthesia. Complications include infection and hemorrhage, but are less common than with cold-knife conization. Damage to the cervical stroma may lead to cervical stenosis or preterm birth associated with cervical incompetence or preterm premature rupture of membranes.

Risk of preterm delivery. Unfortunately, cold-knife conization and LEEP are associated with an increased relative risk of preterm delivery (2.6 and 1.7, respectively). Ablative procedures may not increase the risk of preterm delivery to the same degree, though the risk probably still exists. A deep excisional procedure (cone depth > 10 mm) seems to be an independent risk factor for preterm birth and preterm premature rupture of membranes in subsequent pregnancies. Residual cervical length is also correlated with risk of preterm delivery.

Follow-up. Colposcopic examination should be performed and a cervical smear taken at approximately 4, 10–12, 16–18 and 24 months after treatment. If these assessments are normal, the woman may return to annual screening. The combination of HPV DNA testing for high-risk types and a cytology test at least 6 months after treatment has also been proposed for monitoring. If high-risk HPV DNA is detected, colposcopy should be done. After three negative results have been obtained, annual follow-up is acceptable and should be continued until at least three additional consecutive negative results have been documented.

If the margins on the excised cervical specimen were positive, clinical follow-up with cytology, colposcopy, biopsy and endocervical curettage is appropriate in women who are compliant with frequent monitoring.

Hysterectomy. The indications for hysterectomy as a treatment option for CIN include:
- a conization specimen margin positive for CIN 3, particularly in the setting of completed childbearing or poor compliance with follow-up
- presence of coexistent gynecologic conditions requiring hysterectomy
- patient request
- persistent or recurrent CIN 2 or 3.

Because of the risks associated with hysterectomy, repeated local therapy (e.g. cone biopsy) should also be considered whenever possible.

Recurrent or persistent disease. The rate of recurrent or persistent disease is 5–17%, despite ablative or excisional therapy. Persistent disease has been associated with large lesion size, positive margin status and continuing HPV DNA positivity 6 months or more after treatment.

In retrospective studies biased by ascertainment and treatments, gland involvement has been implicated as a risk factor for recurrent dysplasia; prospective trials show no clinical significance.

HPV vaccination

The two licensed prophylactic HPV vaccines (one bivalent [Cervarix], and one quadrivalent [Gardasil or Silgard]) contain non-infectious virus-like particles (VLPs) which are produced by recombinant technology. The quadrivalent vaccine contains VLPs for HPV types 6, 11, 16 and 18, whereas the bivalent vaccine contains VLPs for HPV types 16 and 18.

Since 2008, the vaccines have become licensed in several countries for use in girls and women. Both vaccines are prophylactic and are administered to prevent infection and consequent disease rather than alter the course of existing HPV infection.

Most countries that recommend the use of these vaccines have programs to vaccinate girls between the ages of 10 and 14 years – before the onset of sexual activity and hence before first exposure to HPV infection. Most countries are also operating a catch-up program targeting different ages (e.g. 17 years, 18 years).

Both vaccines appear to give effective protection against cervical cancer. For example, women in a double-blind placebo-controlled trial (n = 552, mean age 20 years) received the quadrivalent vaccine at months 0, 2 and 6 and were followed up for 3 years. Protection against persistent HPV 16/18 infection occurred in 89% of women who received vaccination and follow-up visits according to protocol, with 100%, 86%, 89% and 100% efficacy for HPV 6, 16, 18 and 11, respectively. After three vaccine doses, seroconversion rates for HPV types 6, 11, 16 and 18 were 94%, 96%, 100% and 76%, respectively, at 36 months. The trial also demonstrated 100% protection against all CIN caused by HPV 6, 11, 16 and 18, and 100% protection against all external genital warts caused by HPV 6 and 11.

In the USA, the Advisory Committee on Immunization Practices and ACOG have recommended that girls and women aged 9–26 years should receive the quadrivalent vaccine. The Centers for Disease Control and Prevention recommend a first dose at age 11–12 years, with catch-up vaccination in those aged 13–26 years if not previously vaccinated. Two further injections are recommended at 2 and 6 months after the initial dose. Including men in the vaccination program is predicted to be more beneficial in reducing HPV infection, and the role of HPV vaccination of men in the prevention of cervical cancer is being considered. HPV vaccination has recently been approved for males.

In the UK, the Department of Health decided to purchase Cervarix (i.e. the bivalent vaccine). There are three factors which are likely to have influenced the Government's decision to adopt Cervarix rather than Gardasil. One of the difficulties with the HPV vaccine is that many have considered it a vaccination against a sexually transmitted infection rather than against a cancer. Cervarix acts against HPV types 16 and 18, which do not cause genital warts but do cause most cases of cervical cancer. Gardasil protects against HPV 16 and 18 but also 6 and 11. HPV 6 and 11 cause around 90% of genital warts and are less common causes of cervical cancer. Therefore, in political terms, it is perhaps easier to 'sell' a vaccine which is for cancer only rather than for a sexually transmitted infection per se. The second factor that has probably influenced the Government is cost. Cervarix is somewhat cheaper than Gardasil. The third factor which may have influenced matters is the data published in the *Lancet*, which showed significant cross-protection against precancerous lesions not containing HPV type 16 and/or 18 as the vaccine provides protection against HPV 31, 33 and 45. This may translate into approximately 11% to 16% extra protection against disease.

The HPV vaccines represent a major advance in the prevention of cervical cancer. Vaccination does not, however, currently replace the need for cervical screening.

Management of invasive carcinoma

In general, a woman presenting with invasive carcinoma to a primary care physician is referred for colposcopy, because the physician taking a cervical smear recognizes that the cervix appears abnormal and makes an immediate referral. Occasionally, referral is made when the cervix looks macroscopically normal, but the smear is suggestive of malignancy. The patient may also be referred if the smear is suggestive of CIN 3 with a macroscopically normal cervix and, on colposcopy, a microinvasive tumor is detected. Eventually, a referral is made to a gynecologic oncologist. The worst method of detection is when a woman develops symptoms (e.g. intermenstrual or postcoital bleeding), is referred and the disease detected. This eventuality is, mercifully, becoming rarer because of the increasing effectiveness and reach of screening programs.

Staging. Historically, staging has been carried out before surgery, but this can under- or overestimate the stage of disease (Table 1.7). The relatively poor sensitivity and specificity of clinical staging has led many to suggest that staging should be surgical. The debate is largely semantic as treatment is never determined by formal staging alone. Currently, treatment recommendations are based on the best possible pretreatment disease assessment even if the most up-to-date methods are not part of official staging. Any lack of concordance in findings from staging investigations should lead to the more advanced stage being selected.

International Federation of Gynecology and Obstetrics (FIGO) guidelines describe the following examinations as useful, but not mandatory, for establishing the stage of disease:
- palpation and inspection of the primary tumor
- palpation of groin and supraclavicular lymph nodes
- colposcopy
- endocervical curettage
- conization
- hysteroscopy

TABLE 1.7

Staging of cervical cancer

	Overstage (%)	Understage (%)	Correct (%)
Stage IB	14.5	19.0	66.5
Stage II	33.5	21.0	45.5

- cystoscopy
- proctoscopy
- intravenous pyelogram
- plain radiographic examination of the lungs and bones.

The American Joint Committee on Cancer developed a parallel tumor–node–metastasis (TNM) classification system, based upon the same preoperative staging information as the FIGO system. The 'T' stages correspond to the FIGO stages with the exception of stage IVB. The findings of surgical/pathological evaluation can be recorded simply as a final pathological disease stage (pTNM), but should not be used to change the clinical stage. As always, treatment is based not on staging, but on the best assessment of disease extent using all possible tests available. For example, computed tomography (CT), positron emission tomography-CT (PET-CT) and magnetic resonance imaging (MRI) are usually performed to determine lymphadenopathy and parametrial spread, respectively, although these are not technically included in the FIGO staging system; Figure 1.6).

MRI is particularly recommended for:
- tumors with a transverse diameter greater than 2 cm
- endocervical or infiltrative tumors that cannot be accurately evaluated clinically
- women in whom clinical examination is difficult, such as those who have other uterine lesions such as leiomyomas, or who are pregnant.

PET is a metabolic imaging technique based on the increased glucose metabolism in tumors. Glucose analog 2-[18F]fluoro-2-deoxy-D-glucose (FDG) is the most common agent used for PET imaging. FDG-PET is very helpful to detect extrapelvic metastasis and metastatic lymphadenopathy in women with advanced cervical cancer.

Other preoperative tests. Women requiring a radical hysterectomy (see later sections) should have, in addition to the staging investigations:
- full blood cell count
- blood group and matched packed cells
- urea and electrolytes
- liver function tests
- CT or PET-CT

Figure 1.6 FIGO staging of cervical cancer.

Stage I   The carcinoma is strictly confined to the cervix; extension to the
                 uterine corpus should be disregarded

    IA   Preclinical carcinomas of the cervix (i.e. those diagnosed by
                 microscopy only). All gross lesions even with superficial invasion
                 are stage IB. Invasion is limited to measured stromal invasion with
                 a maximum depth of 5 mm and no wider than 7 mm on a single
                 slide. Measurement of the depth of invasion should be from the
                 base of the epithelium, either surface or glandular, from which it
                 originates. Vascular space involvement, either venous or
                 lymphatic, should not alter the staging but be reported separately

    IA1   Minimal microscopically evident stromal invasion. The stromal
                 invasion is no more than 3 mm deep and no more than 7 mm in
                 diameter

    IA2   Lesions detected microscopically that can be measured. The
                 measured invasion of the stroma is deeper than 3 mm but no
                 greater than 5 mm, and the diameter is no wider than 7 mm

    IB   Clinical lesions confined to the cervix, or preclinical lesions
                 greater than stage IA

    IB1   Clinical lesions ≤ 4 cm in size

    IB2   Clinical lesions > 4 cm in size

Stage II   Involvement of the vagina (except the lower third) or infiltration
                 of the parametrium. No involvement of the pelvic sidewall

    IIA   Involvement of the upper two-thirds of the vagina, but not out
                 to the parametria

    IIA1   Tumors ≤ 4 cm in size

    IIA2   Tumors > 4 cm in size

    IIB   Infiltration of the parametrium, but not out to the sidewall

Stage III   Involvement of the lower third of the vagina. Extension to the
                 pelvic sidewall. On rectal examination there is no cancer-free
                 space between the tumor and the pelvic sidewall. All cases with
                 a hydronephrosis or non-functioning kidney should be included,
                 unless this is known to be attributable to another cause

    IIIA   Involvement of the lower third of the vagina, but not out to the
                 pelvic sidewall if the parametrium is involved

    IIIB   Extension onto the pelvic sidewall and/or hydronephrosis or non-
                 functional kidney

Stage IV   Extension of the carcinoma beyond the reproductive tract

    IVA   Involvement of the mucosa of the bladder or rectum

    IVB   Distant metastasis or disease outside the true pelvis

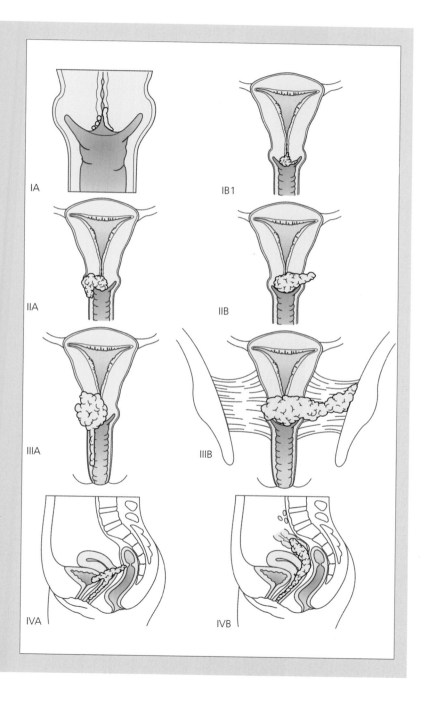

- MRI
- chest X-ray
- ECG
- ureteric visualization (e.g. CT with contrast or MRI from pelvis to kidneys)
- prophylactic antibiotics
- thromboembolic prophylaxis: sequential compression stockings and a heparin preparation.

Management according to stage

Stage IA1, defined as minimal microscopic invasion (< 3 mm) and a small tumor volume (< 7 mm width), with no lymphovascular permeation, can be treated with local therapy in women wishing to retain their reproductive potential. Complete local excision of the lesion is possible because these tumor characteristics define a lesion with minimum metastatic risk.

Many gynecologic oncologists opt for hysterectomy as standard care for well- or moderately differentiated adenocarcinoma of the cervix. Lymph node metastases are rare and the risk of relapse after simple hysterectomy or conization is extremely low.

A woman with early microinvasive adenocarcinoma, no lymph–vascular space invasion (LVSI) and negative cone margins who wishes to preserve her fertility should be extensively counseled regarding the inability to exclude occult invasive disease. Cone biopsy and trachelectomy are treatment options that avoid hysterectomy.

Stage IA2, defined as lesions greater than 3 mm but less than 5 mm in depth, and less than 7 mm in width, can be treated effectively by modified radical trachelectomy/hysterectomy combined with pelvic node dissection. The incidence of pelvic lymph node involvement is 3–4%. In a medically unfit woman, intracavitary radiation (brachytherapy) may be used as an alternative. Laparoscopic or robotic lymph node dissection and vaginal radical trachelectomy or abdominal trachelectomy with lymph node dissection are fertility-sparing approaches.

Microinvasive squamous cervical cancer and microinvasive adenocarcinoma of the cervix are generally treated similarly. However, the glandular lesions are sometimes multifocal. As a result, adenocarcinomas may need more extensive surgical treatment than a similar squamous lesion.

Neuroendocrine tumors of the cervix are rare but have a tendency for early metastasis to bone and brain. Brain imaging, PET and bone scans are often requested for pretreatment assessment. There is no consensus for the treatment of early neuroendocrine tumors of the cervix. A multimodal approach, including surgery, radiotherapy and chemotherapy, should be considered. However, because neuroendocrine tumors are likely to have early occult metastases, neoadjuvant chemotherapy may be preferred for measurable lesions before definitive surgery or radiotherapy.

Modified radical hysterectomy for stage IA2 cervical cancer involves removing the cervix, uterus, uterine artery at the level where it crosses the ureter, upper third of the vagina, medial parametrium and the external and internal iliac and obturator nodes. The para-aortic and common iliac nodes may also be removed.

An alternative to surgery is concurrent chemotherapy and radiotherapy (chemoradiotherapy). The rationale for using slightly lower doses of chemotherapy with radiotherapy is to increase the sensitivity of the tumor to the effect of radiation and to eradicate microscopic systemic disease. Cisplatin has been shown to be a good radiation-sensitizing chemotherapy agent.

Stage IB. Radical hysterectomy or chemoradiotherapy are options for women with larger tumors, up to 4 cm in the greatest dimension (stage IB1). Survival rates with the two approaches are considered equivalent. The treatment recommendations are usually based on the lesion size, extent of infiltration of the cervix with tumor, histological subtype, comorbidities, and physician and patient preference. For instance, a younger woman may prefer surgery to avoid ovarian failure and the vaginal fibrosis associated with high-dose curative radiotherapy.

Adenocarcinoma is more likely than squamous cell carcinoma to spread to the ovaries. Not withstanding this, the ovaries do not need to be removed in early squamous cell cervical cancer or early adenocarcinoma. As the extent of the disease increases, so too does the risk of occult ovarian metastatic disease. Age and reproductive history must be considered in determining the status of the ovaries. If they are not removed during surgery, they should be placed in the paracolic gutters to avoid damage from possible postoperative adjuvant radiotherapy. Postmenopausal women should have their ovaries removed.

If the probability of needing postoperative adjuvant therapy is estimated preoperatively at above 40%, a shift towards recommending chemoradiotherapy is acceptable. Radical surgery with radiotherapy does not appear to improve survival but may have greater morbidity than either treatment alone. For lesions larger than 4 cm, the general preference in North America is for concurrent chemotherapy and radiotherapy. Neoadjuvant chemotherapy followed by surgery is also a reasonable option. Up to 80% of women with stage IB2 disease treated with radical hysterectomy require postoperative adjuvant radiotherapy. Women with positive nodes should be given further therapy with chemoradiotherapy.

Stage II. Women with locally advanced cervical squamous cell cancer (greater than stage IIA disease) are best treated with primary radiotherapy (external beam plus brachytherapy) and concomitant chemotherapy. Nodal involvement, particularly the para-aortic nodes, is the most important adverse prognostic factor, reducing survival by 50%. The available data support a 30–50% reduction in the risk of death from cervical cancer for women with locally advanced disease undergoing radiotherapy and concomitant cisplatin-based chemotherapy compared with radiotherapy alone. Weekly cisplatin, 40 mg/m^2, is used because of its more favorable toxicity profile. The benefit of chemotherapy in combination with extended field radiotherapy in women with positive para-aortic nodes has been reported. Neoadjuvant chemotherapy followed by surgery may also be considered in certain women; several single chemotherapy agents and combination regimens are active in metastatic cervical cancer or recurrences not amenable to local therapy (cisplatin is the most active single agent).

Stages III and IV. Stage III disease is usually treated with chemotherapy as a sensitizer and concomitant radiotherapy. Short-term ureteral stenting or other interventions may be needed until potentially curative therapy is completed.

Treatment of advanced IVB cervical cancer is mostly palliative. Surgery may also be useful in carefully selected patients with isolated pulmonary metastases. Radiotherapy may be useful to palliate the symptoms of pelvic pain or bleeding from advanced disease. Rare complete responses and cures have been reported with chemotherapy alone in advanced cervical cancer.

Chemotherapy. Around 30% of stage IVB or recurrent cancers respond to cisplatin. Median survival is 4–8 months. Ifosfamide, paclitaxel, vinorelbine and topotecan are other single agents used in cervical cancer. Combining topotecan with cisplatin gives a response rate superior to that achieved with cisplatin alone. The combination of paclitaxel and cisplatin has also shown greater response rates than those achieved with either agent singly.

It is important to consider quality of life implications when selecting any therapy, but these are particularly important when recommending chemotherapy. Careful attention should be paid to potential toxicity. Radiotherapy can reduce the pain from metastases at the bone, brain and lymph nodes. New targeted chemotherapy agents are being investigated. In general, adding agents can increase the response rate but may not always improve overall survival. Unfortunately, there is also more toxicity with multi-agent chemotherapeutic regimens.

Surgery. Radical hysterectomy is a challenging operation that involves removing:

- the uterine body, uterine artery and surrounding parametria at its origin from the superior vesical or internal iliac artery
- the entire length and width of the cardinal ligament, cervix and upper third of the vagina
- the paracervical, obturator, presacral, internal, external and common iliac nodes, and in some cases the para-aortic nodes (Figure 1.7).

Current research on sentinel node biopsy is designed to create the evidence base to support its use in preference to pelvic lymphadenectomy. However, at the time of writing, sentinel node biopsy cannot replace 'therapeutic' lymphadenectomy as the results so far are highly variable.

Radical hysterectomy can be performed abdominally, with a mid-line or a low transverse incision (modified Cherny's or Maylard incision), or

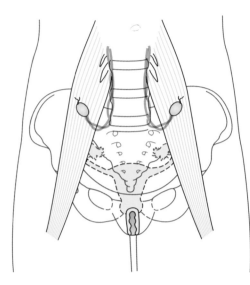

Figure 1.7 Radical hysterectomy showing removal of uterus, cervix, parametrium, upper third of the vagina and lymph nodes. The ovaries are attached post-hysterectomy to the psoas muscle intraabdominally.

vaginally. Laparoscopic and robotic-assisted techniques can be used. The route of hysterectomy depends on the woman and physician's preference, body shape and comorbidities.

Preservation of fertility. For women wishing to preserve fertility, laparoscopic or robotic lymphadenectomy can be performed with a radical trachelectomy, in which a vaginal approach is used to remove the cervix (Figure 1.8). Alternatively, radical trachelectomy can be performed via an abdominal route. A recent review paper reported the morbidity associated with radical vaginal trachelectomy to be low, with a tumor recurrence rate of 5% and a mortality of 3%. The current literature indicates no difference between the rates of recurrence with this technique and with radical hysterectomy when proper selection criteria are used.

Radiotherapy. The two main modalities of irradiation are external pelvic beam and brachytherapy (placement of radioactive sources at a short distance from the intended target).

External beam radiotherapy (EBRT) is used to treat the whole pelvis (including the parametria), pelvic and para-aortic nodes. EBRT can shrink bulky endocervical tumors, improve tumor geometry by

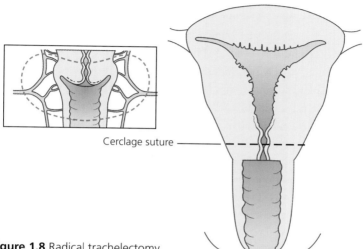

Figure 1.8 Radical trachelectomy.

Cerclage suture

shrinking exocervical tumors, and sterilize the paracentral and nodal area. The pelvic field should include the common iliac, external iliac, internal iliac, obturator and sacral nodes as well as the cervical disease. Curative treatment of cervical cancer usually includes a combination of external pelvic irradiation and brachytherapy, though EBRT can be used alone. Conformal treatment plans, e.g. intensity-modulated radiotherapy, may reduce toxicity to the surrounding tissue.

Brachytherapy. The intracavitary sources irradiate the cervix, vagina and medial parametrium. Used as a sole treatment, brachytherapy involves inserting radioactive material high into the vagina. The procedure is not painful. It is important that appropriate dosing is administered to the central tumor and the pelvic sidewall nodes. The delivered dose is usually calculated at radiotherapy points known as A and B. Point A is situated 2 cm from the midline of the cervical canal, 2 cm cephalad to the ectocervix, and is used relative to the central tumor, while point B is 3 cm to the side of point A (Figure 1.9). Point B and the overlying tissue are important relative to nodal tissue.

Brachytherapy is usually delivered using afterloading applicators that have been inserted into the uterine cavity and vagina. Intrauterine tandem and vaginal ovoids produce a pear-shaped radiation distribution, delivering a high dose of radiation to the cervix and paracervical tissues, and a lower dose to the bladder and rectum. Intracavitary radiotherapy using a low-dose-rate system usually delivers 40–60 cGy per hour to point A. High-dose-rate systems deliver doses at more than 100 cGy per minute to point A. The procedure does not require hospitalization. Studies have shown similar survival and complication rates with low-dose- and high-dose-rate brachytherapy in early cervical cancer. Positive para-aortic lymph nodes can be treated by EBRT. The superior border is usually 'extended' 3 cm above the highest positive node at the level of T12. Timely completion of radiotherapy is essential for a good outcome and it should generally be achieved within 56 days of diagnosis. The use of epoetin or darbepoetin during chemoradiotherapy can maintain hemoglobin levels at 100–120 g/L. Excessive use of erythrocyte-stimulating agents is associated with increased mortality.

Post-treatment follow-up. In the USA, the National Comprehensive Cancer Network suggests clinical evaluation be done every 3 months in year 1, every 4 months in year 2, every 6 months in years 3–5 and then annually. An annual chest X-ray or other imaging modality, including CT or PET, may be necessary as clinically indicated. The clinical evaluation should include a systematic history, a physical examination

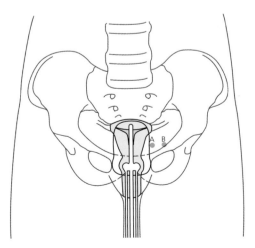

Figure 1.9
Radiotherapy points A and B to treat cervical cancer.

paying particular attention to the supraclavicular and inguinal lymph nodes, a rectovaginal and abdominal examination, and cervical cytology. Asymptomatic disease detected on PET-CT may be treated for cure and extended survival.

Follow-up is similar in the UK, but scans are performed less frequently.

Prognosis. A woman's prognosis is determined by stage, nodal status, tumor volume, depth of cervical stromal invasion, LVSI and, to a lesser extent, histological type and grade. An overview of the prognosis according to cancer stage is shown in Table 1.8. In general, cervical squamous carcinoma has a better prognosis than adenosquamous carcinoma, stage for stage. In addition, adenocarcinoma tends to be diagnosed later and therefore at a more advanced stage, which worsens the prognosis.

Recurrent disease. Although most women with cervical cancer can expect to be cured, initial therapy will be unsuccessful for some, particularly those with advanced disease, and they will face multiple battles with their disease. The disease stage is the most accurate predictor of recurrence. The sites of distant metastases reported include lung (21%), bone (16%), para-aortic nodes (11%), abdominal cavity (8%) and supraclavicular nodes (7%).

Recurrences usually occur within 2 years of initial treatment. Localized central pelvic recurrence, a disease-free interval greater than

TABLE 1.8

Five-year cure rates for cervical carcinoma

Stage	Cure rate
I	85–98%
IIA	75–85%
IIB	65%
IIIA	45%
IIIB	35%
IV	15%

6 months, recurrence less than 3 cm in diameter, and no sidewall fixation are considered favorable prognostic factors for successful salvage treatment. Curative surgery for recurrent disease (pelvic exenteration) is indicated for women who develop a central recurrence (including vaginal apex) without sidewall involvement after primary chemoradiotherapy or after surgery followed by chemoradiotherapy. Non-central recurrence may be managed by laterally extended exenterative procedures. Intraoperative radiotherapy, either with teletherapy or brachytherapy (after loaded devices or permanent implants), may be considered for women with unresectable cancer who have previously received radiotherapy.

Key points – cervical cancer

- Cervical cancer is a disease associated with chronic infection by oncogenic types of human papillomavirus (HPV).
- HPV types 16, 18, 45, 31 or 33 are present in 88% of squamous cancers.
- The progression of all grades of cervical intraepithelial neoplasia to invasive cancer is 1.7%.
- The rate of recurrence or persistence of severe cervical dysplasia is 5–17% despite therapy with any of the excisional or ablative techniques.
- Staging is performed clinically.
- Fertility-sparing surgery is feasible: vaginal trachelectomy for tumors less than 2 cm in diameter; and abdominal trachelectomy for tumors greater than 2 cm in diameter.
- Surgery is preferred for most stage IB1 or smaller cancers.
- Radiotherapy with concurrent low-dose chemotherapy is preferred for localized tumors IB2 to IVA.

Key references

Covens A, Shaw P, Murphy J et al. Is radical trachelectomy a safe alternative to radical hysterectomy for patients with stage IA-B carcinoma of the cervix? *Cancer* 1999;86:2273–9.

Human papillomavirus testing for triage of women with cytologic evidence of low-grade squamous intraepithelial lesions: baseline data from a randomized trial. The Atypical Squamous Cells of Undetermined Significance/Low-Grade Squamous Intraepithelial Lesions Triage Study (ALTS) Group. *J Natl Cancer Inst* 2000;92:397–402.

Keys HM, Bundy BN, Stehman FB et al. Cisplatin, radiation, and adjuvant hysterectomy compared with radiation and adjuvant hysterectomy for bulky stage IB cervical carcinoma. *N Engl J Med* 1999;340:1154–61. Erratum in: *N Engl J Med* 1999;341:708.

Mao C, Koutsky LA, Ault K et al. Efficacy of human papillomavirus-16 vaccine to prevent cervical intraepithelial neoplasia: a randomized controlled trial. *Obstet Gynecol* 2006;107:18–27.

Paavonen J, Naud P, Salmerón J et al. Efficacy of human papillomavirus (HPV)-16/18 AS04-adjuvanted vaccine against cervical infection and precancer caused by oncogenic HPV types (PATRICIA): final analysis of a double-blind, randomised study in young women. *Lancet* 2009;374:301–14.

Peters WA 3rd, Liu PY, Barrett RJ 2nd et al. Concurrent chemotherapy and pelvic radiation therapy compared with pelvic radiation therapy alone as adjuvant therapy after radical surgery in high-risk early-stage cancer of the cervix. *J Clin Oncol* 2000;18:1606–13.

Rose PG, Bundy BN, Watkins EB et al. Concurrent cisplatin-based radiotherapy and chemotherapy for locally advanced cervical cancer. *N Engl J Med* 1999;340:1144–53. Erratum in: *N Engl J Med* 1999; 341:708.

Saslow D Runowicz C, Solomon D et al. American Cancer Society guideline for the early detection of cervical neoplasia and cancer. *CA Cancer J Clin* 2002;52: 342–62.

Schiffman M, Solomon D. Findings to date from the ASCUS-LSIL triage study (ALTS). *Arch Pathol Lab Med* 2003;127:946–9.

Schorge JO, Knowles LM, Lea JS. Adenocarcinoma of the cervix. *Curr Treat Options Oncol* 2004;5: 119–27.

Smith JR, Boyle DC, Corless DJ et al. Abdominal radical trachelectomy: a new surgical technique for the conservative management of cervical carcinoma. *Br J Obstet Gynaecol* 1997;104:1196–200.

Solomon D, Davey D, Kurman R et al. The 2001 Bethesda System: terminology for reporting results of cervical cytology. *JAMA* 2002;287: 2114–9.

Stanley M. HPV vaccines. *Best Pract Res Clin Obstet Gynaecol* 2006;20:279–93.

Ungár L, Pálfalvi L, Hogg R et al. Abdominal radical trachelectomy: a fertility-preserving option for women with early cervical cancer. *BJOG* 2005;112:366–9.

Wright TC, Gagnon S, Richart RM, Ferenczy A. Treatment of cervical intraepithelial neoplasia using the loop electrosurgical excision procedure. *Obstet Gynecol* 1992; 79:173–8.

Wright TC, Schiffman M, Solomon D et al. Interim guidance for the use of human papillomavirus DNA testing as an adjunct to cervical cytology for screening. *Obstet Gynecol* 2004;103:304–9.

Primary cancer of the vagina constitutes 0.3% of all malignant neoplasms of the female genital tract. The risk factors for pre-invasive and invasive squamous cell vaginal carcinoma are the same as for cervical neoplasia: multiple sexual partners over a lifetime, early age at first intercourse and smoking. Although in-utero exposure to diethylstilbestrol is a risk factor, the estimated cumulative lifetime incidence of vaginal clear cell adenocarcinoma following exposure is low (< 1 in 1000).

Most vaginal carcinomas are secondary, arising from primary cancer in the cervix, endometrium or rectum. Less likely primary sites include the colon, ovary and vulva. About one-third of women with primary vaginal cancer have a history of in situ or cervical cancer treated within 5 years prior to the diagnosis of vaginal cancer. If vaginal carcinoma develops more than 5 years after a prior cervical cancer diagnosis, it is considered a new primary lesion.

Diagnosis

The presenting symptoms include:
- painless vaginal bleeding, either postmenopausal or postcoital
- watery, blood-tinged or malodorous vaginal discharge
- vaginal mass
- urinary symptoms
- gastrointestinal complaints.

The posterior wall of the upper one-third of the vagina is the most common site of vaginal carcinoma, and the lesion can appear as a mass, a plaque or an ulcer. Most of the tumors are squamous cell carcinomas, but melanoma, sarcoma and adenocarcinoma including clear cell, have been reported.

Diagnosis can be difficult as vaginal tumors tend to be multicentric and may be hidden behind the blades of the speculum. If a woman presents with an abnormal Pap smear and no gross cervical abnormality, vaginal colposcopy with acetic acid and Lugol's iodine should be performed. Definitive diagnosis is by biopsy.

The staging system used for vaginal carcinoma is shown in Table 2.1.

Vaginal melanoma is rare and occurs mostly in Caucasian women. The lesions are usually located in the distal part of the vagina on the anterior wall.

Age at onset. The average age at which vaginal squamous cell carcinoma develops is 60 years, though age at onset varies widely.

TABLE 2.1

Clinical staging of malignant tumors of the vagina

Staging system

AJCC*	FIGO†	Characteristics
Tx		Primary tumor cannot be assessed
Tis	0	Carcinoma in situ (intraepithelial)
Invasive carcinoma		
T1	I	Confined to vaginal mucosa
T2	II	Submucosal infiltration into parametrium, not extending out to pelvic wall
	IIA‡	Subvaginal infiltration, not into parametrium
	IIB‡	Parametrial infiltration, not extending to pelvic wall
T3	III	Tumor extending to pelvic wall
T4, any N	IVA	Tumor invades mucosa of bladder or rectum or extends outside true pelvis
Any T, any N, M1	IVB	Distant metastatic disease

*2002 American Joint Committee on Cancer (AJCC) primary tumor (T) stage.
†International Federation of Gynecology and Obstetrics (FIGO) stage.
‡Proposed subdivision for stage II lesions.
Used with the permission of the American Joint Committee on Cancer (AJCC), Chicago, Illinois, USA. The original source for this material is the *AJCC Cancer Staging Manual*, 6th edn. New York: Springer, 2002.

In 10% of cases, primary vaginal cancers are adenocarcinomas. The risk is highest in young and very old women, but squamous cell carcinoma is still the most common type affecting all age categories. The peak age at which diethylstilbestrol-related clear cell vaginal adenocarcinoma occurs is 19 years.

Patterns of spread include:

- direct extension to pelvic structures
- hematogenous dissemination to distant organs, including lungs, liver and bone
- lymphatic spread to the pelvic, inguinal and para-aortic lymph nodes.

The upper vagina drains initially into the pelvic nodes and then the para-aortic nodes, while the lymphatics of the distal one-third of the vagina drain first into the inguinal and femoral nodes, and secondarily into the pelvic nodes.

Treatment

Because vaginal cancer is rare, there is no consensus for treatment. Treatment must be tailored to disease stage, site of vaginal lesion and maintenance of a functional vagina.

Surgery has a limited role. Women with stage I disease involving the upper posterior vagina require radical hysterectomy (if uterus is in situ), partial vaginectomy and bilateral pelvic lymphadenectomy. Primary total pelvic exenteration can be recommended to women with stage IVA disease if a rectovaginal or vesicovaginal fistula is present. Total pelvic exenteration can also be offered to women with a central recurrence after chemoradiotherapy.

Radiotherapy is the main treatment. Superficial lesions can be treated with brachytherapy alone. External beam radiation, with or without intracavitary or interstitial brachytherapy, is the usual treatment for stage I lesions greater than 2 cm in diameter and all stage II–IV disease. Radiotherapy to the groin nodes is recommended if the lower third of the vagina is involved. The concurrent use of radiation-sensitizing low doses of cisplatin and/or 5-fluorouracil is appropriate (as it is in cervical and some vulvar malignancies).

Vaginal melanoma. The successful use of wide local excision followed by high-dose radiation fractions to the pelvis (> 400 cGy) has been reported recently for vaginal melanoma.

The best prognostic factor for vaginal melanoma is the size of the lesion. Unfortunately, the overall prognosis is usually poor. Treatment with interferon α-2b is under investigation. Research into cutaneous melanoma may provide additional options in the future.

Complications. Rectovaginal or vesicovaginal fistulas, rectal and vaginal strictures, radiation cystitis and proctitis and, rarely, vaginal necrosis are the main complications of radiotherapy, and sometimes surgical, treatment of vaginal cancer. Continuation of intercourse is encouraged throughout radiotherapy to protect women from vaginal stenosis. In women not sexually active or for whom intercourse is temporarily painful, use of a vaginal dilator with topical estrogen has been suggested.

Prognosis
The stage at the time of presentation, including the size and the depth of tumor infiltration, is the most important variable affecting prognosis. The overall 5-year survival rate for vaginal cancer is about 50%. Survival from stage I disease is high (> 85%).

Key points – vaginal cancer

- Vaginal intraepithelial neoplasia usually precedes vaginal cancer.
- As it is often diagnosed late, vaginal cancer has a poor prognosis.

Key references

Beller U, Sideri M, Maisonneuve P et al. Carcinoma of the vagina. *J Epidemiol Biostat* 2001;6:141–52.

Herbst AL, Ulfelder H, Poskanzer DC. Adenocarcinoma of the vagina. Association of maternal stilbestrol therapy with tumor appearance in young women. *N Engl J Med* 1971;284:878–81.

Endometrial carcinoma

Adenocarcinoma of the endometrium is the most common gynecologic malignancy in North America, and the fourth most common malignancy in women overall. In the USA, over 41 000 women were estimated to develop endometrial cancer in 2008, with 7400 deaths. The cumulative lifetime risk of developing endometrial cancer is 2.6%. The prevalence is lower in the UK, but is rising in line with the increase in obesity.

On a conceptual level, two models of endometrial cancer exist, those related to, and those unrelated to, estrogen stimulation. The two models have different epidemiological and prognostic profiles.

Type I endometrial carcinoma, which accounts for up to 80% of all endometrial carcinoma, is estrogen-related. It is usually a low-grade endometrioid tumor associated with atypical endometrial hyperplasia. The risk factors, which are generally associated with excessive endogenous estrogen, are:

- obesity
- nulliparity
- anovulatory cycles
- estrogen-secreting tumors
- early age at menarche
- late menopause.
  Exogenous sources of excess estrogen include:
- estrogen replacement therapy
- tamoxifen
- a diet containing high amounts of fat (particularly animal fat).

Indirect risk factors include diabetes, hypertension and hereditary risk of cancer. It is not clear whether hypertension alone is responsible for enhancing the risk of endometrial cancer or if the risk is related to the fact that hypertensive women are also generally obese. Similarly, the association with diabetes may be explained mostly by obesity, though insulin can increase the levels of sex hormones and growth factors, and has direct mitogenic effects on endometrial tissue.

Exogenous estrogen. Use of exogenous estrogen is reportedly associated with a 3.1–15-fold increase in endometrial carcinoma, with degree of risk relating to both estrogen dose and duration of use. However, much of the increase in risk may relate to a diagnostic bias prompted by evaluation of symptomatic uterine bleeding formerly associated with relatively high-dose unopposed estrogen therapy. No woman developed endometrial cancer in the oft-cited Postmenopausal Estrogen/Progestin Interventions (PEPI) trial, a 3-year study of unopposed estrogen involving 875 healthy postmenopausal women (45–64 years of age).

Endometrial carcinoma is less aggressive in hormone users, but some investigators have found an increased risk of metastasis. Progestin can reduce the excess risk of endometrial hyperplasia and carcinoma.

Polycystic ovary syndrome (PCOS). The hormonal imbalance that occurs in PCOS can result in prolonged stimulation of uterine cells by estrogen, resulting in endometrial hyperplasia and, in some cases, endometrial cancer. PCOS is often seen in obese women as part of the metabolic syndrome in which adrenal precursors are converted to estrone and estradiol by adipose cells.

Higher body mass index (BMI) is a risk factor for developing endometrial cancer at a younger age (sometimes presenting at age < 45 years). Mortality from endometrial cancer in those with the highest BMI (≥ 40 kg/m^2) exceeds that in women of normal weight. Alterations in the concentration of insulin-like growth factor and its binding proteins, and the increased likelihood of insulin resistance and PCOS may contribute to the increased risk of endometrial cancer in obese women.

Hyperinsulinemia, insulin resistance and insulin-like growth factors play a role in endometrial proliferation and the development of endometrial cancer. Correlation with higher levels of circulating estrogen and androgen, and lower levels of sex hormone binding globulin have been reported in postmenopausal women with endometrial cancer. The involvement of many of these factors may be mediated by the interaction between the α and β estrogen receptors.

Tamoxifen is a variable competitive inhibitor of estrogen binding to estrogen α and β receptors that has partial agonist and antagonist activity. It has been linked to the development of endometrial pathology, including uterine sarcoma. It increases the risk of endometrial cancer two- to three-fold, but the absolute attributable risk is small given the low annual incidence of endometrial cancer. For example, a two-fold relative increase in cancer risk typically represents only one additional cancer for every 1000 women treated. Among women with breast cancer who developed a subsequent endometrial cancer, those treated with tamoxifen were reported to have higher proportions of aggressive endometrial cancers, such as carcinosarcoma and papillary serous cancer.

Genetic factors. It has been reported that women with a history of breast cancer who develop endometrial cancer may have a significantly higher proportion of serous tumors than women with no history of breast cancer. Consistent with this observation, carriers of mutations in *BRCA1* have also been reported to be at an increased risk of uterine cancer.

Type II endometrial carcinomas are not estrogen-dependent. Women tend to present with higher-grade tumors, such as papillary serous, clear cell or poorly differentiated tumors. The profile of women with this type of endometrial cancer differs from that of women with type I. Affected women are often multiparous and older than women with estrogen-related endometrioid tumors. They have a variable prevalence of obesity, diabetes and hypertension. The incidence is also higher in white women. Late diagnosis, higher stage and a higher proportion of poorly differentiated types result in a higher overall mortality. For type II cancers, the prognosis in non-white women may be even worse than for white women.

Epidemiology. Most women with endometrial cancer are in their early sixties, though 25% of cases occur in premenopausal women, with 5–10% occurring in women under 40. Obesity, nulliparity, hypertension and diabetes are more prevalent in young women with well-differentiated pathological types. There is also a higher incidence of synchronous primary ovarian cancers reported in young women with endometrial cancer.

The risk of endometrial cancer decreases with:
- use of combined oral contraception
- smoking, which stimulates hepatic metabolism of estrogens
- increased occupational or recreational physical activity.

Stopping estrogen therapy can reverse most endometrial hyperplasias without further treatment.

The risk factors for endometrial cancer are summarized in Table 3.1.

Genetic alterations. Specific genetic alterations have been reported in endometrial cancer. Mutations in the *PTEN* tumor suppressor gene on chromosome 10q are seen in 30–50% of endometrial cancers. *PTEN* encodes a phosphatase that inhibits the activity of cellular kinases. A further 5% of endometrial cancers are in women with a family history

TABLE 3.1

Risk factors for endometrial carcinoma

Factor	Risk ratio
Combined oral contraceptive pill	0.3–0.5
Smoking	0.5
Obesity	
overweight by 9–22.5 kg (20–50 lb)	3
overweight by > 22.5 kg (50 lb)	10
Nulliparity	
compared with +1 child	2
compared with +5 children	3
Late menopause	
age > 52 years versus < 49 years	2.4
Unopposed estrogen replacement therapy without a progestational agent	10–20
Diabetes	2.8
Tamoxifen	4

Modified from DiSaia PJ, Creasman WT. *Clinical Gynecologic Oncology*, 7th edn. St Louis: Mosby, 2007.

of hereditary non-polyposis colorectal cancer (HNPCC). This reflects germline mutations in DNA mismatch repair (MMR) genes. Women with HNPCC have alterations in the MMR genes *MSH2*, *MSH6*, *MLH1* or, less commonly, *PMS1* and *PMS2*.

Accumulation of genetic mutations happens throughout the genome, but specifically in repetitive DNA sequences called microsatellites, leading to microsatellite instability. Silencing MMR genes through promoter methylation (i.e. somatic mutations of MMR) leads to an increased risk of endometrial cancer. The risk of developing endometrial cancer in HNPCC ranges from 20% to 60%. The cancers associated with HNPCC have earlier onset than sporadic endometrial cancers with de novo acquired mutations. Other sites at increased risk of neoplasms in these families include the ovary, stomach, small bowel, hepatobiliary system and renal pelvis or ureter.

Inactivation of the *p53* tumor suppressor gene is among the most common genetic events in type II endometrial cancer. Other genetic aberrations noted mostly in type II endometrial cancers involve:

- the *CDC4* gene, which is involved in regulating cyclin E expression during cell cycle progression
- the *ER-2/neu* receptor tyrosine kinase gene (possibly amplification of oncogenes with resultant overproduction of the corresponding protein)
- fms oncogene that encodes a tyrosine kinase which serves as a receptor for macrophage-colony stimulating factor (possibly through amplification and overproduction as before).

Diagnosis. Currently, it is not possible to make a rational case for a population-based screening program for endometrial cancer. Fortunately, in most large series, 75% of women are diagnosed as stage I, with 11% at stage II, 11% at stage III and 3% at stage IV. In postmenopausal women, the disease usually presents early as postmenopausal bleeding. Premenopausal women usually present with menstrual irregularity – irregular or heavy vaginal bleeding. The remaining women with endometrial carcinoma, approximately 20%, are diagnosed as a result of abnormal endometrial cells seen on cervical smear. The smear is not, however, an appropriate routine method for detection. Women who should be investigated for endometrial hyperplasia and cancer are listed in Table 3.2.

Endometrial sampling. Postmenopausal bleeding must always be investigated by endometrial sampling (a woman is considered to be postmenopausal when she has not had a period for 1 year). The development of equipment and techniques for outpatient endometrial biopsy has generally replaced the need for the traditional dilatation and curettage (D&C) carried out under either general anesthesia or intravenous analgesia and paracervical block. Histopathology of endometrial specimens taken by biopsy has an excellent correlation with the D&C specimen.

Currently, endometrial assessment tends to be performed either in a clinic with an aspiration biopsy (Figure 3.1) plus transvaginal ultrasound (TVUS) to determine endometrial thickness, or by hysteroscopy with a biopsy (Figure 3.2). Outpatient hysteroscopy can be carried out under paracervical block anesthesia. Hysteroscopy and D&C can be done under sedation or with general or spinal anesthesia. The woman should be advised that it is normal to have some mild cramping and spotting or vaginal bleeding for a few days after

TABLE 3.2

Characteristics of women who should be evaluated for endometrial hyperplasia or cancer

- Over 40 years of age with abnormal uterine bleeding
- Under 40 years of age with abnormal uterine bleeding and risk factors (e.g. chronic anovulation, obesity, tamoxifen use, diabetes, family history of endometrial/ovarian/breast/colon cancer)
- Abnormal uterine bleeding has not responded to medical treatment
- Uterus in situ, receiving unopposed high-dose estrogen replacement therapy
- Atypical glandular cells on cervical cytology
- Endometrial cells on cervical cytology if ≥ 40 years of age
- Those with hereditary non-polyposis colorectal cancer syndrome, starting at age 35 years

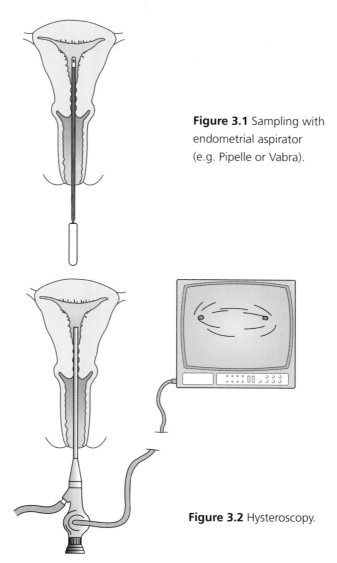

Figure 3.1 Sampling with endometrial aspirator (e.g. Pipelle or Vabra).

Figure 3.2 Hysteroscopy.

endometrial biopsy. Pain relief may be needed, though aspirin may increase the risk of bleeding.

The endometrial thickness threshold of below 3–5 mm may be useful to exclude endometrial cancer in women with a low pre-test probability of endometrial cancer. It does not help to predict who has endometrial cancer (i.e. it has a low positive predictive value).

55

The American Cancer Society recommends annual screening by endometrial biopsy, initiated by the age of 35 years, for women:
- known to carry HNPCC-associated mutations
- with a family member known to carry one of these mutations
- from families with a predisposition to colon cancer in the absence of genetic testing.

Ultrasound-based investigation. Most women with postmenopausal bleeding do not have endometrial cancer. TVUS is accepted as a screening tool to identify those at highest risk of malignancy. An endometrial thickness equal to or more than 4 mm requires endometrial sampling in a postmenopausal woman with bleeding. TVUS is also recommended when the diagnosis is unclear after biopsy, and for those women with a relative contraindication to proceeding to hysteroscopy with D&C. Hysteroscopy with D&C is not suitable for the primary evaluation of abnormal bleeding as it does not give a definitive diagnosis, is painful and has a high cost.

Pathology. Histologically, endometrial carcinoma falls into the following subtypes:
- endometrioid carcinoma (most common)
- villoglandular adenocarcinoma
- adenocarcinoma with benign squamous element, squamous metaplasia or squamous differentiation (adenoacanthoma)
- adenosquamous carcinoma
- papillary serous adenocarcinoma
- clear cell carcinoma
- squamous cell carcinoma
- undifferentiated carcinoma.

Carcinoma of the corpus should be graded according to the degree of differentiation of the adenocarcinoma:
- G1: $\leq 5\%$ non-squamous or non-morular solid growth pattern
- G2: 6–50% non-squamous or non-morular solid growth pattern
- G3: > 50% non-squamous or non-morular solid growth pattern.

Hysteroscopy with D&C is indicated after a non-diagnostic outpatient endometrial biopsy in women at risk of endometrial carcinoma. It is also indicated despite a benign histology from an outpatient biopsy in women with persistent abnormal uterine bleeding, insufficient tissue for analysis, or cervical stenosis preventing outpatient endometrial biopsy. Many practitioners prefer to go straight to hysteroscopy with D&C.

Although hysteroscopy has a role in the diagnosis of some cases of endometrial cancer, the impact of hysteroscopy on prognosis is unclear. An increase in positive malignant cytology after endometrial cancer diagnosed on hysteroscopy has been reported.

Intraperitoneal spillage of the fluid used in the procedure along with endometrial cancer cells from the fallopian tubes is possible, but may not be an independent risk factor. The prognosis may be worsened because the cytology results reflect other, more important, prognostic factors such as grade.

Surgery is usually undertaken once the histological diagnosis has been made. Surgical staging of the cancer is the most accurate method in most women (Figure 3.3).

Vaginal hysterectomy alone has been proposed in women not fit for extensive surgery because of comorbid conditions. Radiotherapy may be an appropriate first-line therapy for a very frail woman.

Preoperative management. The following preoperative investigations and management should be considered:
- full blood count
- urea and electrolytes
- liver function tests
- chest X-ray
- CT of the abdomen and pelvis
- MRI (the best radiographic modality for assessing myometrial invasion and cervical involvement, but not useful if surgery is to be performed regardless of the result)
- measurement of cancer antigen 125 (CA125), a clinically useful marker for predicting extrauterine spread of endometrial cancer
- ECG
- blood grouping and autologous collection or cross-matching
- thromboembolic and antibiotic prophylaxis.

Fertility preservation. As the average age of first conception increases in society at large, so an increasing number of women

Figure 3.3 FIGO staging of endometrial carcinoma.

Stage I

IA   Tumor limited to the endometrium or invasion of less than half of the myometrium

IB   Invasion of equal to or more than half of the myometrium

Stage II

    Cervical stromal invasion

Stage III

IIIA   Tumor invades serosa and/or adenexae

IIIB   Metastases to vagina, parametrium or pelvic peritoneum

IIIC   Metastases to retroperitoneal lymph nodes

IIIC1   Positive pelvic node

IIIC2   Positive para-aortic node

Stage IV

IVA   Tumor invasion of the bladder and/or bowel mucosa

IVB   Distant metastases including intra-abdominal and/or inguinal lymph nodes

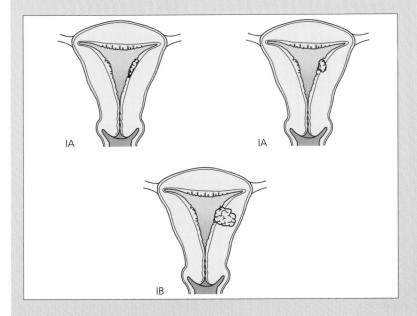

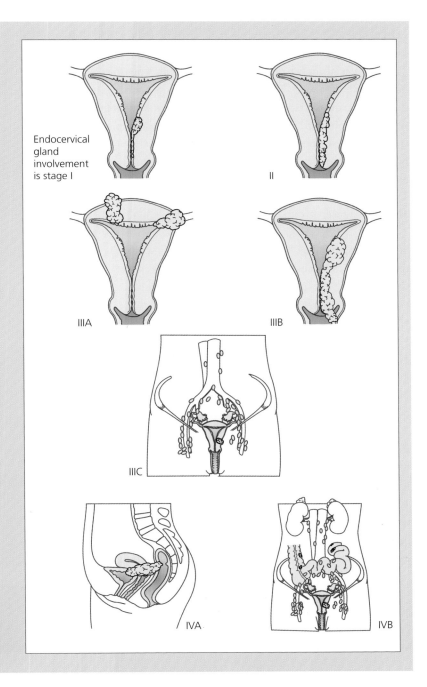

Endocervical gland involvement is stage I

with cancer will wish to preserve their fertility. Up to 15% of women with endometrial cancer will be of reproductive age (i.e. < 40 years).

Endometrial cancer can be treated with oral progestins if there is no evidence of spread. Tests should include endocervical curettage, pelvic MRI, measurement of CA125, Pap smear and an assessment of fertility potential. If all the investigations indicate no evidence of spread, grade 1 tumor and normal fertility, then 3–9 months of hormone therapy is reasonable. Repeat outpatient endometrial aspiration and brush sampling, and MRI at 3-monthly intervals. The progesterone intrauterine device and aromatase inhibitors may also have a role.

Surgical staging. The Society of Gynecologic Oncologists and ACOG recommend that most women with endometrial cancer undergo complete surgical staging. The US approach includes:
- washings for cytological evaluation
- hysterectomy
- bilateral salpingo-oophorectomy (BSO)
- pelvic and para-aortic nodal sampling (see below)
- biopsy of any suspicious area.

Management in the UK is slightly less aggressive, with nodal sampling omitted for some women (see below).

Radical hysterectomy is sometimes considered when the cervix is involved. Peritoneal fluid is collected, or normal saline is placed intraperitoneally and then aspirated for cytological evaluation. About 15% of women have positive peritoneal cytology. To exclude the possibility of adnexal micrometastases or synchronous tumors, BSO is recommended, as the ovaries are a site of estrogen production. Ovarian preservation can be considered in well-counseled young women with low-risk disease.

In the USA, there is currently a preference for lymph node sampling in all medically fit women. This is based on the presumption that knowledge of lymph node status will affect the selection of adjuvant treatment. Because it is not possible to accurately predict the risk of lymph node spread preoperatively or intraoperatively, many advocate staging all endometrial cancers. In the UK, lymph node sampling is performed only in the event of enlarged nodes.

High risk of nodal disease. A high risk of nodal disease is indicated by:
- high-grade histology (including serous, clear-cell and poorly differentiated carcinomas)
- myometrial invasion of more than 50%
- large tumor (> 2 cm in diameter)
- lower uterine or cervical involvement
- enlarged lymph nodes
- gross extrauterine disease.

Whether nodal sampling or lymphadenectomy and extended para-aortic node dissection should be performed is controversial; whichever procedure is selected, it should be performed by an experienced surgeon. Regardless of the extent of surgery, the status of the pelvic and para-aortic lymph nodes should always be assessed by inspection and palpation. Unfortunately, up to 20% of women report lymphedema affecting the lower extremities after pelvic lymphadenectomy, particularly if pelvic radiotherapy has been used after surgery.

High presurgical risk of metastasis (e.g. those with elevated CA125, grade 3 cancer or high-risk histology) may not require lymph node sampling because adjuvant therapy is already indicated. In women at very high risk, the only indication for lymph node removal would be the theoretical treatment effect for the lymphadenectomy (see above).

Management according to risk of recurrence

Risk of recurrence depends on surgical stage, tumor grade and histological subtype (Table 3.3). Adjuvant treatment after surgical staging is recommended for women at intermediate and high risk of recurrence.

Another way of considering the risk of recurrence is to class the disease as organ-confined or extrauterine.

Low risk. Women with stage I grade 1 or 2, or IA grade 1 histology confined to the uterine fundus, with no involvement of the

TABLE 3.3

Risk of recurrence in women with endometrial cancer

Low risk (5%)

- Stage I, grade 1 or 2 with invasion of the inner third or less of the myometrium

Intermediate risk (10%)

- Stage I, grade 1 or 2 with invasion of the middle or deep third of the myometrium
- Stage II, invasion of the cervix or isthmus and no involvement of the lymphovascular space

High risk (14–42%)

- Grade 3 disease with > 50% myometrial invasion
- Stage IIB, III or IV disease
- All high-risk histologies, e.g. clear cell and serous carcinomas

lymphovascular space and no evidence of lymph node metastases, require no further treatment after complete surgical staging. Adjuvant hormonal treatment with progestins has no significant benefit.

High intermediate risk of pelvic recurrence. The efficacy of and the indications for adjuvant radiotherapy following surgery remain controversial. A Gynecologic Oncology Group study defined a subgroup of women at high intermediate risk of pelvic recurrence as:

- women with moderate to poorly differentiated tumor, lymphovascular invasion and invasion of the outer third of the myometrium
- age 50 or older with any two of the factors listed in the first bullet point
- age 70 or older with any risk factor listed in the first bullet point. The study concluded that adjuvant radiotherapy in early stage intermediate risk endometrial carcinoma decreases the risk of

recurrence, but that it should be limited to women whose risk factors fit a definition of high intermediate risk.

High risk. In women with upper abdominal disease (stage III or IV), adjuvant chemotherapy has a survival advantage over radiotherapy. Chemotherapy has a survival advantage in early-stage high-risk disease, e.g. grade 3, deeply invasive cancer. Women with high-risk histologies (e.g. sarcoma) are also likely to benefit from adjuvant chemotherapy. Because radiotherapy has been used traditionally, some oncologists recommend a 'sandwich' regimen, in which the proven beneficial chemotherapy is given before and after pelvic irradiation.

Adjuvant treatment

Chemotherapy. *Progestins.* Numerous studies show progestins to have minimal efficacy when used as adjuvant therapy. However, some women with recurrent disease do benefit, and there is little associated morbidity. The women most likely to benefit are those with grade 1 tumors positive for estrogen and progestin receptors. About one-third of recurrent cancers will respond. The preferred regimen is either medroxyprogesterone acetate (Depo-Provera), 500 mg intramuscularly at weekly intervals, or oral medroxyprogesterone acetate (Provera), 200 mg daily.

Other agents. Recurrent disease responds to other agents, such as cisplatin. Compared with single-agent regimens, combination regimens are associated with higher response rates, greater toxicity and smaller increases in some important outcomes, but they have little additional effect on overall survival.

Women with high-risk or advanced extrauterine disease. Adjuvant chemotherapy is recommended for women with advanced extrauterine disease. The most effective regimen and duration of treatment have not been defined. The reported response rates of various combination regimens that include doxorubicin and/or a platinum-containing drug with or without cyclophosphamide are slightly higher than those reported for the respective monotherapies. Study data show a response rate above 50% with the combination of carboplatin and paclitaxel. Several randomized trials involving women with high-risk histology and women with advanced stage disease have shown chemotherapy to have a meaningful survival advantage over radiotherapy.

Radiotherapy has been used as an adjuvant for more than half a century. Unfortunately, several randomized controlled trials have failed to show a survival advantage for radiotherapy.

Toxicity. Pelvic radiotherapy is more likely than brachytherapy to be harmful to the gastrointestinal tract. Intensity-modulated radiotherapy (IMRT) applies the prescribed dose to the volume of the target tissues in three dimensions. IMRT may decrease acute and chronic toxic effects on the bowel.

Prognosis

The prognosis in women with endometrial cancer depends on disease stage and intra- and extrauterine factors, which include:
- histological type
- tumor grade
- myometrial invasion
- isthmus–cervix extension
- invasion of the vascular space
- adnexal metastasis
- intraperitoneal spread
- positive peritoneal cytology
- pelvic node metastasis
- aortic node metastasis.

In addition to the risk of recurrence (see Table 3.3), the prognosis is related to tumor receptor status and the DNA ploidy of the tumor.

Survival rates at 5 years are:
- 80% for stage I
- 70% for stage II
- 45% for stage III
- 16% for stage IV.

Recurrent disease

Most recurrences of endometrial cancer occur within the first 3 years of diagnosis, with 40% of women having local recurrence in the vaginal vault or pelvis. The remaining 60% whose cancer recurs have distant recurrence in the upper abdomen or lung. Recurrence is less likely in areas previously irradiated. Consequently, distant metastatic recurrent disease is more likely after adjuvant radiotherapy.

The US National Comprehensive Cancer Network recommends that post-treatment surveillance includes:

- physical examination every 3–6 months for 2 years, and annually thereafter
- vaginal cytology every 6 months for 2 years, and annually thereafter
- measurement of serum CA125 at each visit for women whose initial level was elevated.

UK practice is similar, but it does not include vaginal cytology, as recurrences typically present with vaginal bleeding.

Women with recurrent disease must be considered for palliative treatment or treatment intended to cure.

Vaginal cuff or pelvic recurrence should be treated with radiotherapy. Isolated vaginal location and lack of previous radiotherapy are associated with prolonged survival following salvage radiotherapy. If the residual disease is thicker than 3–5 mm, a combination of external beam radiotherapy (EBRT) to a total dose of 45–50 Gy and interstitial brachytherapy is recommended. For apical lesions, a vaginal template under laparoscopic guidance is used to deliver a total EBRT dose of 75–85 Gy. Radiotherapy can be used for the salvage of non-central local or regional recurrences.

Central recurrence after primary surgery and radiotherapy. Pelvic exenteration is associated with a high operative morbidity and poor overall survival, but it remains the only potentially curative option for these women.

Metastatic disease outside a single radiation field. Systemic treatment can be used. Hormone therapy (progestins, selective estrogen-receptor modulators or aromatase inhibitors) is an option for women with advanced hormone-receptor-positive endometrial cancer.

Uterine sarcoma

Uterine sarcomas are a rare form of aggressive cancer that can arise from the endometrium or the myometrium. Sarcomas comprise 1% of gynecologic malignancies and fewer than 5% of all cancers of the uterus. The overall survival rate is under 50%. Surgical resection is the mainstay of the treatment. Response to adjuvant chemotherapy or radiotherapy is poor. A FIGO staging system is used to grade uterine sarcomas, which include uterine malignant mixed mullerian tumor or carcinosarcoma, leiomyosarcoma, endometrial stromal sarcoma and adenosarcoma (Table 3.4).

Carcinosarcoma, which accounts for 43% of all sarcomas, is usually detected in women over 40 years of age. African-American ethnicity, a history of pelvic radiotherapy and tamoxifen use increase the risk of uterine carcinosarcoma.

TABLE 3.4

FIGO staging system for uterine sarcoma

Stage I: limited to uterus

- IA   < 5 cm
- IB   ≥ 5 cm

Stage II: tumor extends to the pelvis

- IIA   adnexa
- IIB   other pelvic tissue

Stage III: invades abdominal tissue

- IIIA   1 site
- IIIB   >1 site
- IIIC   pelvic or para-aortic nodes

Stage IV

- IVA   bladder or rectum
- IVB   distant metastasis

Carcinosarcomas often form bulky polyploid masses that extend into or through the endocervical canal. Their aggressiveness is usually caused by the carcinomatous component (endometrioid, serous or clear cell); metastasis occurs mostly to the lungs and omentum. The 5-year survival rate is lower than 20%. Surgical debulking is still recommended. Staging is not necessary as it is reasonable to treat all women with a definitive preoperative diagnosis of carcinosarcoma with adjuvant therapy.

Radiotherapy combined with chemotherapy is a good approach. Ifosfamide with or without cisplatin, and carboplatin plus paclitaxel have been used in combination with radiotherapy. The current treatments are associated with a poor response and high recurrence rates.

Leiomyosarcoma accounts for more than one-third of uterine sarcomas. The average age at diagnosis is 53 years. Endometrial biopsy has a low detection rate for leiomyosarcoma and as few as 15% of women are diagnosed preoperatively.

Clinical presentation. Leiomyosarcoma appears clinically as a large (> 10 cm) solitary mass with infiltration into the adjacent myometrium. Lung metastasis can occur early, and preoperative thoracic CT imaging is recommended if the diagnosis is known.

Histology. Hypercellularity, coagulative tumor cell necrosis, abundant mitoses (≥ 10–20 per 10 high-power fields), atypical mitoses, cytological atypia and infiltrative borders are noted.

Surgical staging for uterine leiomyosarcoma is the same as for endometrial carcinoma. The pelvic and para-aortic nodes are not typically involved at the time of primary surgery, so the importance of lymph node dissection is unclear. Staging is unnecessary if adjuvant therapy is to be used regardless of stage, but may still be useful for determining prognosis.

Treatment. Combined treatment with radiotherapy and chemotherapy should be considered, even for women with disease confined to the uterus. At the very least, adjuvant chemotherapy should be strongly considered.

If extrauterine disease is present, chemotherapy and palliative radiotherapy for symptomatic tumors can be considered. In some cases, tumor debulking can be undertaken after response to treatment. The cure rate for women with disease confined to the uterus is 20–60%; it depends on the success of the primary resection. The recurrence rate is about 70% in stage I and II disease. Radiotherapy has been shown to reduce the pelvic recurrence rate by 50%, but there is no survival benefit.

Chemotherapeutic agents, such as ifosfamide, doxorubicin, gemcitabine and liposomal doxorubicin, have been used. The risk of progressive disease in women treated with chemotherapy is as high as 80%. If local recurrence occurs, surgical resection can be considered, but cure is unlikely.

Endometrial stromal sarcoma accounts for fewer than 5% of uterine sarcomas. Most women with endometrial stromal sarcoma are premenopausal and present with bleeding and pain. Two histological subtypes have previously been used – low grade and high grade – but the current literature uses the term 'undifferentiated uterine sarcoma' rather than high-grade endometrial stromal sarcoma. In low-grade endometrial stromal sarcoma, proliferative endometrial stromal cells are present, and are described as worm-like plugs of tumor within the vascular or lymphatic channels of the myometrium. Cytological atypia is mild to moderate, with fewer than 10 mitoses per 10 high-power fields, and cells often express estrogen and progesterone receptors.

Surgical staging is recommended. Hormone therapy should be offered, and radiotherapy considered, if estrogen and progesterone receptors are positive. Radiotherapy alone is recommended in the absence of positive receptors. Treatment with progestins has a 33–45% response rate in women with low-grade endometrial stromal sarcoma. The effects of medroxyprogesterone acetate, estrogen receptor modulators, progesterone receptor modulators (mifepristone) and aromatase inhibitors are being explored. Radiotherapy is recommended for early stage endometrial stromal sarcoma. Combination treatment is an option for women with hormone-receptor-positive endometrial stromal sarcoma.

Adenosarcoma has a benign epithelial component mixed with a malignant sarcomatous element. It accounts for 25% of all uterine sarcomas. The average age at diagnosis is 58, and women present with excessive vaginal bleeding and pelvic pain. The tumor may protrude from the cervical os. Adenosarcoma is typically considered to be a low-grade malignancy, and local recurrence is 20%. Typically, a recurrence after an initial diagnosis of adenosarcoma is pure sarcoma.

Surgical staging is recommended for adenosarcoma and hormone therapy is an option. Radiotherapy and chemotherapy are used, particularly where there is sarcomatous overgrowth (i.e. high-grade pure sarcoma occupying 25% or more of the tumor volume). The prognosis is poor for a woman with sarcomatous overgrowth.

Key points – uterine cancer

- In general, endometrial cancers are diagnosed early, and hence they usually have a good prognosis.
- Fertility-sparing treatment with progestins may be possible in stage IA disease.
- Randomized trial data on the therapeutic value of lymphadenectomy are conflicting and have led to differences in routine between the USA and Europe.
- Radiotherapy is the traditional adjuvant treatment.
- Chemotherapy has a proven survival advantage as adjuvant treatment.

Key references

American College of Obstetricians and Gynecologists Practice Bulletin, Clinical Management Guidelines for Obstetrician-gynecologists, number 65, August 2005: management of endometrial cancer. *Obstet Gynecol* 2005;106:413–25.

Bancher-Todesca D, Neunteufel W, Williams KE et al. Influence of postoperative treatment on survival in patients with uterine papillary serous carcinoma. *Gynecol Oncol* 1998;71: 344–7.

Ben-Shachar I, Pavelka J, Cohn DE et al. Surgical staging for patients presenting with grade 1 endometrial carcinoma. *Obstet Gynecol* 2005;105:487–93.

Bland AE, Calingaert B, Secord AA et al. Relationship between tamoxifen use and high risk endometrial cancer histologic types. *Gynecol Oncol* 2009;112:150–4.

Bristow RE, Zahurak ML, Alexander CJ, Zellars RC, Montz FJ. FIGO stage IIIC endometrial carcinoma: resection of macroscopic nodal disease and other determinants of survival. *Int J Gynecol Cancer* 2003;13:664–72.

Cragun JM, Havrilesky LJ, Calingaert B et al. Retrospective analysis of selective lymphadenectomy in apparent early-stage endometrial cancer. *J Clin Oncol* 2005;23:3668–75.

Farhi DC, Nosanchuk J, Silverberg SG. Endometrial adenocarcinoma in women under 25 years of age. *Obstet Gynecol* 1986;68:741–5.

Fleming GF, Brunetto VL, Cella D et al. Phase III trial of doxorubicin plus cisplatin with or without paclitaxel plus filgrastim in advanced endometrial carcinoma: a Gynecologic Oncology Group Study. *J Clin Oncol* 2004;22:2159–66.

Kadar N, Malfetano JH, Homesley HD. Determinants of survival of surgically staged patients with endometrial carcinoma histologically confined to the uterus: implications for therapy. *Obstet Gynecol* 1992;80:655–9.

Kelly MG, O'Malley D, Hui P et al. Patients with uterine papillary serous cancers may benefit from adjuvant platinum-based chemoradiation. *Gynecol Oncol* 2004;95:469–73.

Keys HM, Roberts JA, Brunetto VL et al. A phase III trial of surgery with or without adjunctive external pelvic radiation therapy in intermediate risk endometrial adenocarcinoma: a Gynecologic Oncology Group study. *Gynecol Oncol* 2004;92:744–51.

Randall ME, Filiaci VL, Muss H et al. Randomized phase III trial of whole-abdominal irradiation versus doxorubicin and cisplatin chemotherapy in advanced endometrial carcinoma: a Gynecologic Oncology Group Study. *J Clin Oncol* 2006;24:36–44.

Cancer of the ovary is the second most common gynecologic cancer – it accounts for 26% of tumors, but 52% of the total mortality. The probability of a newborn girl developing ovarian cancer over the course of her lifetime is 1.4% (i.e. 1 in 70). The lifetime chance of dying from ovarian cancer is 1.05% or 1 in 95.

Ovarian cancer is most common in women aged 55–59 years, but it can occur at any age. The incidence is higher among white women than black women, and it is increasing. This is in contrast to the incidence of breast cancer, which has remained constant, and cervical and endometrial cancers, which have fallen in incidence. The incidence trend may possibly be a reflection of women having smaller families and, with increasing affluence, an increasingly high-fat diet.

Risk factors

Some of the epidemiological risk factors associated with ovarian cancer are shown in Table 4.1. There is also an association with colon, breast and endometrial cancer (all four cancers are associated with high-fat diets).

Exposure to ovarian stimulatory drugs has been linked with ovarian cancer, a finding that is consistent with the observation that factors that suppress ovulation (e.g. pregnancy and the oral contraceptive pill) are protective. However, successfully treated infertility is actually associated with a reduction in the risk of ovarian and endometrial cancer. If there is a causal association, it is not excessive. Certainly, in pursuit of the goal of having a child, a small risk is not unreasonable.

Postmenopausal hormone replacement therapy is reported to be associated with an increased risk of ovarian cancer. The Cancer Prevention Study II, with more than 200 000 postmenopausal women, revealed a two-fold increase in risk of mortality from ovarian cancer if estrogen had been used for more than 10 years. The Women's Health

TABLE 4.1

Risk factors for ovarian cancer

- Nulliparity
- Infertility
- A high-fat diet
- Higher socioeconomic status
- Family history

- Celibacy
- Irradiation of pelvic organs
- Early menarche
- Exposure to talc and asbestos

Initiative study revealed an increased relative risk of developing ovarian cancer with the use of combined hormone replacement therapy. However, the absolute attributable risk was actually quite small (< 1/10 000 women treated). Once a woman has developed ovarian cancer, estrogen therapy does not appear to affect the likelihood of recurrence.

Genetic susceptibility. Hereditary ovarian cancer accounts for 5–10% of all ovarian cancers. Two susceptibility genes for breast and ovarian cancer, *BRCA1* and *BRCA2*, have been determined. The presence of mutations in *BRCA1*, located on chromosome 17, increases the lifetime risk of ovarian cancer by 28–44%. Mutations in *BRCA2*, which is located on chromosome 13, increase the lifetime risk of ovarian cancer by up to 27%.

Mutations in mismatch repair genes increase the risk of ovarian cancer about three-fold. Other genetic mechanisms and genes associated with ovarian cancer include:
- mutation in tumor suppressor genes
- loss of heterozygosity
- p53 mutations
- c-myc
- *ERBB2*
- *AKT2*
- *PIK3C*
- ras mutations (more common in borderline ovarian tumors).

Pathology

Epithelial ovarian cancers may arise from the ovarian surface epithelium or distal fallopian tube. Most remain as a cyst. Exfoliation of ovarian cancer cells into the peritoneum can occur, with extension to the right paracolic gutter and the hemidiaphragm. As a consequence of the circulation of peritoneal fluid, the omentum and all the peritoneal surfaces are at risk of involvement. Ovarian cancer can also spread through the retroperitoneal lymphatic vessels that drain the ovary.

The World Health Organization (WHO) published guidelines on the histological classification of ovarian malignancy in 1973; the broad divisions are shown in Table 4.2. The guidelines were updated in 1999, and another update is in progress. The WHO classification differentiates epithelial tumors into benign, borderline and malignant grades.

TABLE 4.2

Histological classification of ovarian malignancies

I Common epithelial tumors	II Sex cord (gonadal stromal) tumors
(Each type is classified as benign, borderline, malignant)	A Granulosa–stromal cell tumor
A Serous	B Androblastoma; Sertoli–Leydig cell tumor
B Mucinous	C Gynandroblastoma
C Endometrioid	D Unclassified
D Clear cell (mesonephroid)	**III Lipid (lipoid) cell tumors**
E Brenner tumors	**IV Germ cell tumors**
F Mixed epithelial tumors	A Dysgerminoma
G Undifferentiated carcinoma	B Endodermal sinus tumor
H Unclassified epithelial tumors	C Embryonal carcinoma
	D Polyembryoma
	E Choriocarcinoma
	F Teratoma
	G Mixed forms

A borderline tumor has some but not all of the features of cancer including, in varying combinations:

- stratification of the epithelial cells
- apparent detachment of cellular clusters from their sites of origin
- mitotic activity
- nuclear abnormalities intermediate between those of clearly benign or malignant changes.

Obvious stromal invasion must not be present in tumors classified as borderline.

The pathological characteristics of low malignant potential or borderline tumors are a total microinvasive area of less than 10 mm^2 and a depth of invasion of not more than 3 mm.

Screening

Unfortunately, most women with ovarian cancer present when their cancer is advanced, with the result that survival rates are poor. The search for an effective screening test has been hampered by uncertainty over whether a premalignant phase of the disease can be detected. Any test must have a very high specificity and sensitivity because ovarian evaluation is difficult.

To date, research has centered around vaginal examination, ultrasound scanning (including Doppler color flow imaging) and tumor markers, the most prominent of which has been CA125. However, none of these techniques, either alone or in combination, has proven suitable for screening the general population. The relative specificities and sensitivities of each test are shown in Table 4.3. The positive and negative predictive values are most important. Although the sensitivity and specificity may seem favorable, the prevalence of disease limits the interpretations of these values.

Combined approaches. Combining serum markers (e.g. insulin-like growth factor-1, leptin, osteopontin and CA125) can improve the overall accuracy of serum screening and, in theory, be clinically useful. In a high-risk population, the positive and negative predictive values can be helpful.

TABLE 4.3

Potential tests for detecting early stage ovarian cancer

Test	Specificity (%)	Sensitivity at 1 year (%)
CA125	97.0	70
Vaginal examination	97.3	–
Ultrasound	98.0	90
Vaginal examination and ultrasound	99.0	–
Multifactor serum analysis (prolactin, IGF, leptin, CA125, macrophage-inhibiting factor and osteopontin)	99.4	95
CA125 and ultrasound	99.8	70
CA125 and vaginal examination	100	70
CA125, ultrasound and vaginal examination	100	–
HE4	95	90

CA125, cancer antigen 125; IGF, insulin-like growth factor.

In the UK, a large study (approximately 20 000 women) has looked at a sequential combination of serum CA125 measurement and ultrasound in screening for ovarian cancer. The screening protocol had a specificity of 99.9%, a positive predictive value of 26.8%, and an apparent sensitivity of 78.6% and 57.9% at 1- and 2-year follow-up, respectively.

The usefulness of a sonogram is limited by the lack of a premalignant morphologic state that can be imaged.

High-risk women. Approximately 10% of ovarian cancer is genetically inherited. In the UK and the USA, screening using CA125 and ultrasound is now sometimes recommended for women at high risk for ovarian cancer. The risk of developing cancer based on familial incidence has been defined by Lynch (Table 4.4) who has, with others, demonstrated that there is a 'cancer-prone' hereditary non-polyposis colorectal cancer (HNPCC) family. Members of this family have an

TABLE 4.4

Risk of heritable ovarian cancer*

Number of first-degree relatives affected	Relative risk
One	2.5
Two	30

*The background risk is 1 in 70.

increased risk of developing carcinoma of the breast, colon, ovaries and endometrium. However, only risk-reducing surgery (i.e. oophorectomy), and possibly some medical therapies are effective. Screening high-risk women currently leads to documentation of the natural history of ovarian cancer without improved survival. So-called 'sonogram-associated deaths' occur when a woman at high risk of ovarian cancer, who has completed childbearing, is imaged regularly until ovarian cancer develops. Obviously, this is too late for primary prevention.

Management of women at high genetic risk

Oral contraceptive pill. As using oral contraceptives appears to decrease the risk of ovarian cancer in the general population, *BRCA* carriers are encouraged to use the oral contraceptive pill as a chemopreventive agent. However, the data on the increased risk of breast cancer in these carriers are controversial.

Risk-reducing surgery. The incidence of gynecologic cancers is reduced dramatically (by 96%) after risk-reducing prophylactic bilateral salpingo-oophorectomy (BSO). The risk of *BRCA* carriers developing subsequent breast cancer is reduced by 50–80%. The Society of Gynecologic Oncology has made recommendations for prophylactic BSO based on the findings that, for women with *BRCA1* mutations, the risk of ovarian cancer begins to rise in the late 30s and early 40s. For women with *BRCA2* mutations, the risk of ovarian cancer does not begin to rise until around 10 years later (risk is only 2–3% by 50 years of age). So, for women with *BRCA1* mutations, it recommends that risk-reducing BSO be offered after childbearing has finished and only deferred following a careful discussion of the risks and benefits. For women with *BRCA2* mutations, the risk of breast cancer by the age of 50 may be as high as 26–34%, and deferral of BSO until the natural menopause may cause the loss of the substantial protection against breast cancer that the procedure affords.

If risk-reducing surgery is elected, the uterus need not be removed providing a preoperative endometrial biopsy is benign and the family history does not suggest an increased risk of endometrial cancer. Retaining the uterus greatly reduces the risk of the surgery. Both ovaries and as much of the fallopian tubes as possible must be removed because of the small risk of fallopian tube cancer. Many occult cancers are found incidentally during presumed prophylactic BSO – sometimes cancer is present only in the tube. For this reason, the entire specimen should be sectioned every 2–3 mm. Washings should also be sent during prophylactic surgery. Risk-reducing hysterectomy plus BSO should be considered on a case-by-case basis for high-risk women. The risk of developing a primary peritoneal cancer persists after surgery (1–6%).

Diagnosis

A recent study revealed that 95% of women with ovarian cancer did, in fact, have symptoms before they were diagnosed. The most common were abdominal and gastrointestinal complaints, and the least common were pelvic or gynecologic symptoms. The common symptoms, which are vague and non-specific, include:
- abdominal bloating
- changes in bowel function
- constipation
- early satiety
- urinary complaints
- pelvic pressure
- pain.

Physical examination may reveal a pelvic mass, peritoneal intra-abdominal disease or both. CA125 may be elevated, particularly in postmenopausal women. Other tumor markers, such as carcinoembryonic antigen and cancer antigen 19-9 (CA19-9) can also be elevated in ovarian cancer.

Staging

Staging of ovarian cancer can only be carried out surgically, and it is vitally important that a complete staging procedure is always undertaken. Inadequate staging, followed at a later date by adequate staging, has shown that approximately 30% of ovarian cancers are more advanced than they originally seemed. The exception to this approach is for advanced tumors, which may be treated first with chemotherapy and then cytoreduced surgically at a later date.

The staging procedure involves a vertical incision, cytological washings, intact tumor removal, complete abdominal exploration, removal of remaining ovaries, uterus and tubes, omentectomy, lymph node sampling (for apparent early-stage ovarian cancer) and tumor and lymph node debulking for advanced ovarian cancer. Random peritoneal biopsies should be taken: the diaphragm should be included as a sampling site in early ovarian cancer. The FIGO staging for ovarian cancer is shown in Figure 4.1.

Tumors are also graded 1–3, with grade 1 being the least aggressive and grade 3 the most aggressive. The grade affects the prognosis and treatment.

Preoperative management

Preoperative investigations and management may include:

- full blood count, blood typing and, possibly, autologous blood collection or cross-matching
- measurement of urea and electrolytes, CA125, CA19-9 and carcinoembryonic antigen (CEA)
- liver function tests
- serum stored for other tumor markers if required
- pelvic examination and cervical smear
- CT and ultrasound
- bowel preparation may be considered in some cases
- antibiotic prophylaxis and thromboprophylaxis.

Imaging

The inability of current imaging techniques to visualize the peritoneum accurately gives rise to problems with preoperative diagnosis and staging.

While ultrasound is a good technique for detecting ovarian cysts, particularly when augmented with Doppler color flow imaging, it is a poor tool for visualizing nodal disease and peritoneal involvement. In addition, it cannot reliably distinguish between benign and malignant lesions.

CT allows better visualization of the lymph nodes, but it will detect only nodes greater than 1 cm in diameter. CT can also detect liver metastases, ascites and peritoneal involvement, though it is not uncommon for these to be under- or over-diagnosed. Combining CT with a functional study such as PET can increase the accuracy of imaging. In women with a high pre-test probability of cancer (e.g. potentially recurrent disease), this combination can be considered diagnostic.

MRI may be a useful adjunct, but it is subject to similar errors. CT is probably still the best modality for identifying lymph nodes, whereas MRI is better for assessing soft tissue spread. Findings from MRI, CT and ultrasound are rarely sufficient to establish a definitive diagnosis.

Surgery

Unfortunately, with ovarian cancer, it is not possible to predict accurately the stage of disease before laparotomy. An extensive discussion with the woman is required before surgery, based partly on the results of the preparatory investigations.

Postmenopausal women. In a postmenopausal woman with an adnexal mass, it is standard procedure to carry out a hysterectomy, BSO and greater omentectomy. Lymphadenectomy or sampling may also be performed, as may bowel resection if the bowel is involved.

Premenopausal women. The absolute minimum level of investigation includes peritoneal washings, diaphragmatic and paracolic gutter samples and removal of the affected ovary and greater omentum. Suspicious peritoneal lesions should be biopsied and sent for histological investigation. Any palpable lymph nodes should be sampled. Frozen-section analysis can be used intraoperatively to determine whether an ovarian mass is benign, borderline or cancerous.

Figure 4.1 FIGO staging of ovarian cancer

Stage I   Growth limited to the ovaries

    IA   Growth limited to one ovary, no ascites

            No tumor on the external surface, capsule intact

            Tumor present on the external surface and/or capsule ruptured

    IB   Growth limited to both ovaries, no ascites

            No tumor on the external surface, capsule intact

            Tumor present on the external surface and/or capsule ruptured

    IC   Tumor either stage IA or B but with ascites or positive peritoneal washings

Stage II   Growth involving one or both ovaries with pelvic extension

    IIA   Extension and/or metastases to the uterus and/or tubes

    IIB   Extension to other pelvic tissues

    IIC   Tumor either stage IIA or B, but with ascites or positive peritoneal washings

Stage III   Growth involving one or both ovaries with intraperitoneal metastases outside the pelvis and/or positive retroperitoneal or inguinal nodes; or tumor limited to the true pelvis with histologically proven malignant extension to small bowel or omentum; superficial liver metastases

    IIIA   Tumor grossly limited to the true pelvis with negative nodes but with histologically confirmed microscopic seeding of abdominal peritoneal surfaces

    IIIB   Tumor of one or both ovaries; histologically confirmed implants of abdominal peritoneal surfaces, none exceeding 2 cm in diameter; nodes negative

    IIIC   Abdominal implants 2 cm in diameter and/or positive retroperitoneal nodes or inguinal nodes

Stage IV   Growth involving one or both ovaries with distant metastases. If pleural effusion is present, there must be positive cytology to allot a patient to stage IV. Parenchymal liver metastases

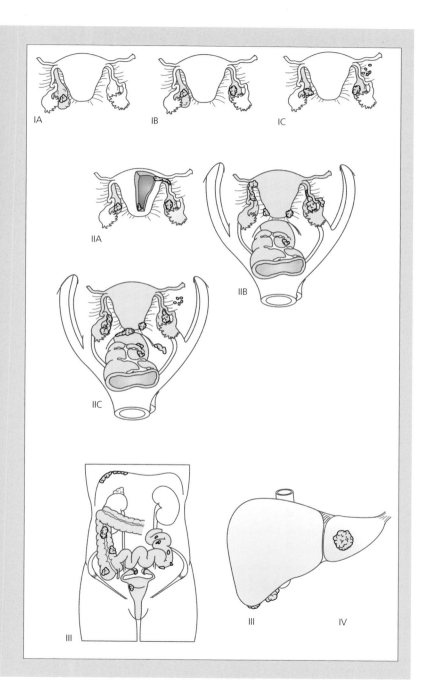

Lymph nodes should only be removed if cancerous. There is a small chance of false-negative results that require repeat laparotomy.

Management of a premenopausal woman wishing to retain her fertility has to be individualized and based on the intraoperative findings. Many women opt to have an oophorectomy and full surgical staging, while retaining the uterus and contralateral tube and ovary. A further laparotomy to remove the other ovary and the uterus can be carried out later if required.

Differentiation between benign and malignant disease is often not possible either at laparotomy or on frozen section, and diagnosis must be confirmed by subsequent permanent section histology. In some women, malignancy is more obvious; but even here (e.g. in the case of pseudomyxoma), benign disease can masquerade as malignancy. Therefore, the gynecologic oncologist should wait for full histology results if in doubt. When invasive disease is confirmed, management must comprise cytoreductive surgery proportional to organ involvement.

Cytoreduction. Surgery aims to reduce the tumor cell volume as much as possible in order to improve chemosensitivity. Removing non-dividing and hypoxic tumor helps reduce the number of chemotherapy cycles required, decreasing the risk of resistant clones developing and enhancing immunologic competence. The ideal outcome is that no macroscopic tumor is visible at the end of the procedure. Failing this, the tumor should be reduced to nodules as small as possible (preferably < 1 cm).

In stage III ovarian cancer, 5-year survival has been reported as:
- 40–70% with microscopic disease
- 30–40% with optimal cytoreduction
- 5% with suboptimal debulking.

'Heroic' surgery that is likely to leave the tumor more than 1 cm or more in diameter is probably best avoided.

Postoperative management

Most ovarian cancers are at stages II, III or IV. Stages IA and IB are manageable by surgery alone, but women with stage IC, II, III or IV ovarian cancer require adjuvant chemotherapy. Postoperative management of stage IA (grade 3) and IB differs between the UK and USA. In the UK, most women are managed individually and on an expectant basis. In contrast, adjuvant chemotherapy is usually used for all grade 3 tumors in the USA. Positive cytology resulting from intraoperative rupture is not desirable, but it is usually not considered an indication for chemotherapy.

Reassessment surgery. Repeat, or 'second-look' reassessment, surgery after chemotherapy was a standard regimen in the late 1970s and 1980s, though the approach was adopted without rigorous evaluation. It is now used in trial protocols and there is some evidence that operating after chemotherapy to achieve tumor shrinkage may be beneficial.

If intraperitoneal chemotherapy ports are needed, many surgeons prefer to place the access device in a second operation during which residual tumor can also be removed. In theory, placing the peritoneal port during a second procedure reduces the risk of port-associated complications.

Secondary tumor debulking can be considered if surgically resectable recurrent disease occurs at least 12 months after chemotherapy has been completed.

Palliative surgery can be considered for relief of bowel obstruction, and can include colostomy, bowel resection, bowel bypass, ileostomy and gastrostomy tube placement.

Chemotherapy

The most significant advances in chemotherapy for ovarian cancer have been the introduction of:

- alkylating agents (1970s)
- platinum-based agents (which extended the median survival for ovarian cancer from 12 to 20 months) (1980s)
- paclitaxel in combination therapy, further extending median survival to 36 months (1990s)
- intraperitoneal chemotherapy.

In general, the platinum-taxane combination is the preferred initial adjuvant regimen for all ovarian cancers requiring chemotherapy; the alternatives are reasonable, however. European data and some US trials have provided support for single-agent platinum compounds. The better toxicity profile makes single-agent carboplatin a more appropriate regimen for some women.

Consolidation or maintenance therapy consists of prolonged treatment (6–12 months) with a lower dose of chemotherapy. This is started after the standard chemotherapy management. It remains controversial as the effect on overall survival is unknown.

Relatively equivalent multidrug regimens can be considered for women with special requirements. Although specific recommendations regarding chemotherapy regimens will undoubtedly change relatively frequently, the platinum-based agents and taxanes will continue to have a principal role in treatment of ovarian cancer, at least in the near future.

Neoadjuvant chemotherapy refers to the administration of chemotherapy before definitive surgery is performed; this approach was introduced for ovarian cancer approximately one decade ago, initially for malnourished women medically unable to tolerate aggressive cytoreductive surgery. Subsequently, neoadjuvant chemotherapy was used for women in whom optimal cytoreductive surgery could not be performed. One potential advantage of neoadjuvant chemotherapy and interval debulking surgery over standard cytoreductive surgery and adjuvant chemotherapy is reduced perioperative morbidity. It also offers a way to avoid aggressive surgery for women with chemoresistant disease, who have a poor outcome regardless of treatment.

Advanced cancers. Compelling evidence now exists to support the use of a taxane combined with a platinum-based agent in the management of advanced (stages III and IV) ovarian cancer. This treatment regimen is superior to previous treatments for tumors that have been debulked optimally (< 1 cm) and suboptimally (> 1 cm), in terms of progression-free survival, overall survival and quality of life. Overall, this combination probably contributes, on average, an extra year of life at a cost of £7200 per life-year gained. Response to second-line treatment in women who have relapsed following first-line treatment depends on the length of the initial remission period – the longer the remission, the better the prognosis.

Intraperitoneal chemotherapy. The US National Cancer Institute has encouraged the use of intraperitoneal chemotherapy following reports of a survival advantage with intraperitoneal chemotherapy compared with intravenous chemotherapy in women with optimally cytoreduced stage III epithelial ovarian cancer. Intraperitoneal chemotherapy is, however, more toxic than intravenous chemotherapy. If intraperitoneal chemotherapy ports are needed, some surgeons prefer to place the access device in a second operation. In theory, placing the peritoneal port during a second procedure reduces the risk of port-associated complications.

Intraperitoneal chemotherapy should be included as part of postoperative adjuvant therapy in most women with cancer at an advanced stage. Drugs with low peritoneal and high peripheral clearance should be used, and suggested agents include paclitaxel, cisplatin and floxuridine (not licensed in the UK).

Currently, intraperitoneal chemotherapy is used less commonly in the UK than in the USA.

Perioperative hyperthermic intraperitoneal chemotherapy may offer a therapeutic advantage over standard intraperitoneal chemotherapy for women with optimal tumor debulking (preferably with no gross residual tumor). At the end of the surgery, while the woman is still anesthetized, an inflow and outflow catheter is temporarily sutured into place and the abdomen sealed. Heated chemotherapy (40–44°C) is circulated for approximately 90 minutes. Simultaneously, the woman is cooled to approximately 35°C. The catheters are then removed and the abdomen closed completely. An alternative method, which can be carried out as an outpatient procedure, simplifies the process by heating the chemotherapy during infusion through a previously placed intraperitoneal port. No outflow catheter is used. No randomized trial data are available for either method.

Response to chemotherapy. Overall response rates to chemotherapy vary significantly. For example, women with disease that progresses during first-line platinum therapy have an approximate response rate of 30% to a second-line regimen. Progression during treatment with a second agent places the woman in an extremely poor prognostic category, with typical response rates of around 15% to third-line agents. In contrast, if a woman has a complete and durable response (e.g. > 1 year to recurrence), response to re-treatment with the same initial regimen can be around 80%.

In-vitro chemopredictive assays. To assist in predicting the response, in-vitro chemopredictive assays are available that expose cultured tumor cells taken from the woman to chemotherapy. Using the in-vitro response to predict the clinical response to chemotherapy can theoretically improve survival, reduce costs and minimize toxicity.

Adjuvant radiotherapy

The role of adjuvant radiotherapy in the treatment of ovarian cancer is unclear. A high rate of intestinal obstruction has been observed with whole-abdomen radiation. Intraperitoneal ^{32}P has been used in the past, but shows no survival benefit over cisplatin.

Recurrent or persistent disease

Recurrent or persistent disease is detected with biochemical (HE4, serum tumor markers), radiographic (CT, PET-CT) and clinical evaluation. Frequent assays for tumor markers such as CA125 do not improve survival and may adversely affect quality of life. In the USA the following schedule is used for clinical evaluation:

- every 3–4 months for 2 years, then
- every 6 months for 3 years, then
- annually.

In the UK, radiographic imaging is performed less often.

Management of recurrent disease is even more variable than the treatment of primary disease. It depends on the time to recurrence, the number of recurrences and the location of the disease.

If relapse occurs 3 months after completing the initial treatment, it is considered platinum-refractory disease. If relapse is within 6 months, it is considered platinum-resistant disease. Platinum-sensitive disease recurs after 6 months. The most common agents used are liposomal doxorubicin, gemcitabine, topotecan, paclitaxel, docetaxel, altretamine (not licensed in the UK), oral etoposide, and platinum-based compounds, such as cisplatin or carboplatin. Different molecular targets such as tyrosine kinase, vascular endothelial growth factor (VEGF), mitogen-activated protein kinase/extracellular signal-regulated kinase (MEK), mammalian target of rapamycin (mTOR) and insulin-like growth factor (IGF) have been investigated, and agents directed at them are becoming part of chemotherapy regimens in every setting. Many phase I trials of new agents are conducted, but few go on to show clinically meaningful benefit in phase III studies.

High-dose chemotherapy with bone marrow transplant is again being evaluated for eradication of minimal residual disease.

Resistance to chemotherapy. Eventually, most ovarian cancers develop resistance to all available chemotherapy agents. However, with sequential treatment, many women can experience a prolonged survival despite multiple recurrences. A shift from attempting to cure recurrent disease with multi-agent regimens to 'palliative' single-agent chemotherapy may reflect a changed perception of ovarian cancer to that of a 'chronic' disease. In women with little chance of cure, intensive multi-agent regimens can lead to resistance relatively quickly. Worse still, multi-agent regimens are more toxic than single-agent treatment, leaving women unable to tolerate re-treatment with a different regimen. In clinical situations with a low pre-test probability of response (i.e. after multiple recurrence), a chemoresistance assay may predict which agents are unlikely to be effective. This information can be used to eliminate useless and potentially toxic chemotherapy selections.

Monoclonal antibodies. Trials of monoclonal antibodies against ovarian cancer-associated antigens in recurrent disease are under way. A humanized monoclonal antibody that targets VEGF has shown an effect when used in combination with other cytotoxic agents. A major side effect is the risk of gastrointestinal perforation during treatment.

Hormone therapy has demonstrated a moderate response in women with recurrent ovarian cancer.

Additional or secondary cytoreductive surgery can benefit women with recurrence following a long disease-free interval. Whether this approach is suitable depends on many factors, including comorbid conditions, anticipated response to chemotherapy and length of disease-free interval. Women with localized disease are the best candidates for re-operation. Certainly, a 5-year disease-free interval warrants additional surgery while 6 months without recurrence does not.

Prognosis

A poor prognosis is associated with clear cell carcinomas of the ovary, increased tumor ploidy, older age and volume of ascites. The prognosis also depends on the stage of the tumor (Table 4.5) and the efficacy of

TABLE 4.5

Survival rates for ovarian cancer

Stage	3-year survival rate (%)	5-year survival rate (%)
I	92.4	89.3
II	73.2	65.5
III	48.9	33.5
IIIA	61.8	45.3
IIIB	54.0	38.6
IIIC	51.2	35.2
IV	30.1	17.9
No stage	41.5	29.5
Total	54.4	43.9

Data from Kosary CL. Cancer of the ovary. In: Gloeckler Ries LA et al., eds. *Survival Among Adults: U.S. SEER Program*, 1988–2001, Patient and Tumor Characteristics. Bethesda: National Cancer Institute, 2007. Available from www.seer.cancer.gov.

the initial debulking procedure. Based on older second-look data, if no grossly visible residual tumor is left after surgery, 80% of women will be in remission at 2 years, while 50% of women left with optimal residual tumor mass (< 1 cm) will be in remission at 2-year follow-up. In contrast, suboptimal debulking (> 2 cm) results in only 20% of women remaining clear of disease at 2 years. Whatever the surgical outcome, treatment with first-line platinum and taxanes has been shown to improve prognosis.

Cancer of the fallopian tubes

Cancer of the fallopian tubes is rare (0.41 per 100 000 women). It is often mistaken for ovarian cancer until laparotomy is performed. The tumor is staged surgically, and the procedure is similar to that used to stage ovarian malignancy. In almost every clinically important parameter, fallopian tube cancer resembles ovarian cancer. A hypothesis has been proposed that early fallopian tube cancer is the precursor to serous ovarian cancer.

Non-epithelial ovarian cancers

Approximately 10% of ovarian cancer is non-epithelial – germ cell tumors and sex cord-stromal tumors account for the greatest proportion. The prognosis tends to be better with non-epithelial than with epithelial ovarian cancers. In part, this reflects an earlier stage at presentation. The serum tumor markers associated with germ cell and sex cord-stromal tumors are shown in Tables 4.6 and 4.7.

Germ cell tumors usually occur between 10 to 30 years of age, and they are more prevalent in Asian and black girls and women. Patients may present with abdominal pain, distension caused by torsion or hemorrhage, vaginal bleeding and precocious puberty, or signs of pregnancy. Tumor growth is rapid, and the girl or woman may experience a sudden onset of pelvic pain from a rapidly enlarging mass that ruptures or undergoes torsion. Preoperative evaluation requires measurement of serum human chorionic gonadotropin (hCG), α-fetoprotein and lactate dehydrogenase (LDH), and renal and liver function tests. CT helps with assessment and to rule out distant

TABLE 4.6

Serum tumor markers in malignant germ cell tumors of the ovary

Histology	Tumor marker		
	AFP	hCG	LDH
Dysgerminoma	−	±	+
Endodermal sinus tumor (yolk sac)	+	−	+
Immature teratoma	±	−	±
Mixed germ cell tumor	±	±	±
Choriocarcinoma	−	+	±
Embryonal cancer	±	+	±
Polyembryoma	±	+	−

AFP, α-fetoprotein; hCG, human chorionic gonadotropin; LDH, lactate dehydrogenase.

TABLE 4.7

Markers secreted by sex cord-stromal tumors of the ovary

	E2	Inhibin B	T	And	DHEA
Thecoma-fibroma	−	−	−	−	−
Granulosa cell	+	+	−	−	−
Sertoli-Leydig	−	±	+	+	−
Gonadoblastoma	±	±	±	±	±

And, androstenedione; DHEA, dihydroepiandrostenedione; E2, estradiol; T, testosterone.

metastasis. When presenting as an emergency, cystectomy or unilateral salpingo-oophorectomy is appropriate pending final pathological diagnosis. Future childbearing should be discussed with the woman.

Dysgerminoma is the most common malignant ovarian germ cell tumor. The tumor is bilateral in 10% of cases. LDH and hCG can be used as tumor markers. Dysgerminoma spreads via the lymphatics, particularly to the higher para-aortic nodes. Fertility-sparing surgical staging can be performed for women yet to complete childbearing and includes:

- oophorectomy
- palpation of the contralateral ovary or biopsy
- unilateral pelvic lymphadenectomy
- para-aortic node sampling
- peritoneal biopsies
- omentectomy.

Full surgical staging, for women who have completed childbearing, includes a hysterectomy and BSO.

Dysgerminomas are sensitive to radiation, but radiotherapy is not the first-line treatment. Systemic chemotherapy is used as an adjuvant treatment for all women except those with stage IA dysgerminoma. Combination therapy using bleomycin, etoposide and cisplatin is reported to be the most effective regimen.

Most recurrences occur within the first year of initial treatment.

Immature teratomas contain tissue from the three germ cell layers: ectoderm, mesoderm and endoderm. Occurrence of immature teratoma is high between the ages of 10 and 20 years. α-Fetoprotein is used as a tumor marker. The grading system (1–3) is based on the degree of differentiation and quantity of immature tissue, which is established histologically. Surgical staging is similar to that for dysgerminoma. Advanced disease requires cytoreductive surgery. Stage IA grade I immature teratoma does not require postoperative chemotherapy; bleomycin, etoposide and cisplatin is the preferred treatment regimen for all other stages and grades.

Endodermal sinus or yolk sac tumors are aggressive cancers common in the first two decades of life. Typically, Schiller-Duval bodies are present; these are small cystic spaces with central glomerulus-like projections with a fibrovascular core. α-Fetoprotein is used as a tumor marker. All girls and women with endodermal sinus tumors are treated with chemotherapy after the surgical staging procedure, which is similar to that used for the other germ cell tumors.

Other malignant germ cell tumors are rare. Measurement of tumor markers is helpful in the diagnosis and follow-up of germ cell malignancies.

Sex cord-stromal tumors derive from the cells surrounding the oocytes, including the cells that produce the ovarian hormones. They account for 5–8% of all ovarian malignancies. In the presence of an adnexal mass on ultrasound, estrogen excess with precocious puberty, abnormal uterine bleeding, endometrial hyperplasia, carcinoma or androgen excess with virilization should raise suspicion of a sex cord-stromal tumor.

Granulosa cell tumor is the most common sex cord-stromal tumor. The mean age at presentation is 52 years. It is considered a low-grade malignancy. The tumor secretes estrogen. Hemoperitoneum can be present. Concurrent, well-differentiated endometrioid cancer is reported in 5–10% of cases.

Two subtypes of granulosa cell tumor are reported: adult and juvenile. The juvenile subtype accounts for only 5% of cases, and typically develops before puberty. Granulosa cells of the adult subtype appear with 'coffee-bean' grooved nuclei. The cells are arranged in small clusters or rosettes around a central cavity, and these constitute the Call-Exner bodies. Adult subtype granulosa cell tumors have a microfollicular pattern, while juvenile subtypes present with a macrofollicular or cystic pattern.

Inhibin B, which is secreted by granulosa cell tumors, can be used as a diagnostic and follow-up tumor marker in postmenopausal women. Premenopausal women have varying levels of inhibin, making it less useful as a marker.

Unilateral salpingo-oophorectomy with staging can be considered for stage IA as a fertility-preserving option. Perioperative endometrial biopsy or dilatation and curettage should be done. The contralateral ovary may be biopsied if clinically indicated.

If preservation of fertility is not important, full surgical staging should be performed.

There are no data to support a survival benefit with postoperative chemotherapy for women with resected disease. However, in advanced disease bleomycin, etoposide and cisplatin is recommended for all women, given the potential for a better long-term survival. The median time to recurrence is 4–6 years.

Sertoli–Leydig cell tumors produce androgens. Clinical virilization is present in 70–85% of women. The mean age at diagnosis is 25 years, with women typically presenting with abdominal pain. The average size of the pelvic mass is 16 cm. Testosterone is used as the tumor marker for diagnosis and follow-up treatment. The surgical approach is the same as that used for granulosa cell tumors. Prognosis is related to the stage and tumor grade (well differentiated, moderately differentiated and poorly differentiated). Chemotherapy is an option for metastatic disease. Bleomycin, etoposide and cisplatin is recommended for advanced Sertoli–Leydig cell tumors.

Sex-cord tumors with annular tubules often produce estradiol and progesterone. Abnormal uterine bleeding may occur. More than 30% of cases are associated with Peutz–Jeghers syndrome. The principles of surgical staging are similar to those for epithelial ovarian cancer.

Other tumor types in this class are mostly benign neoplasms.

Other ovarian tumors include metastatic tumors and sarcoma. Ovarian carcinosarcoma behaves aggressively, and is treated with surgery and chemotherapy.

Key points – ovarian cancer

- Most ovarian cancers are epithelial carcinomas.
- Surgical staging is performed for all stages of disease.
- Optimal primary tumor debulking remains the cornerstone of ovarian cancer management.
- Neoadjuvant chemotherapy followed by interval tumor debulking surgery can be considered for patients with unresectable advanced ovarian cancer or significant morbidities.
- Combination taxane and platinum-based chemotherapy is being used as the first-line treatment for epithelial ovarian cancer.
- Fertility-sparing surgery can be considered for most young patients with non-epithelial ovarian cancer.

Key references

Andersen JE, Zee B, Paul J, Baron B, Pecorelli S. Randomized intergroup trial of cisplatin-paclitaxel versus cisplatin-cyclophosphamide in women with advanced epithelial ovarian cancer: three-year results. *J Natl Cancer Inst* 2000;92:699–708.

Armstrong DK, Bundy B, Wenzel L et al. Intraperitoneal cisplatin and paclitaxel in ovarian cancer. *N Engl J Med* 2006;354:34–43.

Aunobl B, Sanches R, Didier E, Bignon YJ. Major oncogenes and tumor suppressor genes involved in epithelial ovarian cancer (review). *Int J Oncol* 2000;16:567–76.

Burke W, Daly M, Garber J et al. Recommendations for follow-up care of individuals with an inherited predisposition to cancer. II. BRCA1 and BRCA2. Cancer Genetics Studies Consortium. *JAMA* 1997;277:997–1003.

Cannistra SA. Cancer of the ovary. *N Engl J Med* 2004;351:2519–29.

Chemotherapy for advanced ovarian cancer. Advanced Ovarian Cancer Trialists Group. *Cochrane Database Syst Rev* 2000, issue 2. CD001418. www.thecochranelibrary.com

Jacobs I, Davies AP, Bridges J et al. Prevalence screening for ovarian cancer in postmenopausal women by CA 125 measurement and ultrasonography. *BMJ* 1993;306:1030–4.

Morris RT, Gershenson DM, Silva EG, Follen M, Morris M, Wharton JT. Outcome and reproductive function after conservative surgery for borderline ovarian tumors. *Obstet Gynecol* 2000;95:541–7.

Pal T, Permuth-Wey J, Betts JA et al. BRCA1 and BRCA2 mutations account for a large proportion of ovarian carcinoma cases. *Cancer* 2005;104:2807–16.

Schwartz PE. Neoadjuvant chemotherapy for the management of ovarian cancer. *Best Pract Res Clin Obstet Gynaecol* 2002;16:585–96.

Society of Gynecologic Oncologists Clinical Practice Committee Statement on prophylactic salpingo-oophorectomy. *Gynecol Oncol* 2005;98:179–81.

Epidemiology and etiology

Vulvar cancer accounts for 3–5% of all genital tract malignancies in women and its incidence appears to be increasing. It is primarily a disease of the elderly. In many series, over half of women with vulvar cancer are over the age of 70 years. The rising incidence may, therefore, reflect the aging female population. However, it has also been noted that approximately 15% of women with vulvar cancer are under 40 years of age.

The etiology is not as well understood as that of cervical neoplasia, but sexually transmitted diseases (STDs) appear to be involved. There may be an association with recurrent infection with herpes simplex virus (HSV). An association between human papillomavirus (HPV) and vulvar cancer has been shown. Multifocal warty or bowenoid lesions are identified in younger populations and are related to HPV infection. Atrophic lesions such as lichen sclerosis and ulcerative genital disease are also associated with vulvar neoplasia.

The most important risk factor is the presence of vulvar dysplasia or squamous vulvar intraepithelial neoplasia (VIN). Smoking and immunosuppression are also risk factors. Invasive cancer has been reported in 5–30% of VIN excisions.

Pathology

Most lesions are squamous (85%) in origin (Figure 5.1), but all cancers that can affect skin can also affect the vulva. These include melanoma, sarcoma, adenocarcinoma and basal cell carcinoma. In addition, tumors can arise in the Bartholin's glands (< 1%). Verrucous carcinoma is a special variant of the squamous type. Despite achieving a large size, this tumor rarely metastasizes and can be treated with partial radical resection (radiotherapy may induce anaplastic transformation of the lesions, and consequently it is contraindicated). Other rare histologies include: Merkel cell, transitional cell and adenocystic carcinomas; Paget's disease of the vulva; and various sarcomas.

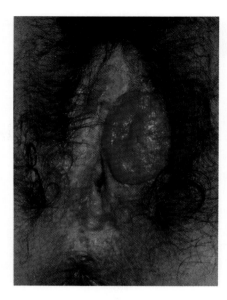

Figure 5.1 Exophytic squamous vulvar carcinoma (4 × 5 cm in size) involving left labia minor and majora.

Clinical presentation

Lesions probably develop, over a prolonged period of time, from VIN. VIN may be asymptomatic or may be associated with pruritus. Many lesions arise de novo. A wart-like growth may occur, and this can be confused with HPV-related condyloma acuminatum. Women with frank carcinoma may have either a cauliflower-like growth or ulceration, which can be asymptomatic or associated with pruritus, pain, bleeding and a foul smell. On questioning, many women will admit to having symptoms over many months and, unfortunately, many may also have been treated medically without biopsy or even examination for many months before referral. The golden rule with vulvar lesions is: if in any doubt, carry out a biopsy.

Pattern of spread includes direct extension to the vagina, urethra, clitoris and/or anus, with or without lymphatic embolization to the regional lymph nodes. Lymph node involvement can occur early in the course of disease, while hematogenous spread occurs late.

Ulcerative lesions. Any ulcerative lesion suspected of having an infectious etiology (Figure 5.2) should be investigated thoroughly

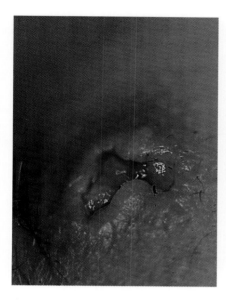

Figure 5.2 A herpetic ulcer on a background of HIV infection. Clinically, this was highly suspicious of carcinoma.

by an STD specialist. If tests are negative or the lesion does not respond promptly to medical management, a biopsy should be performed. Similarly, a biopsy should be taken from any growths on the vulva. If vulvar warts are being treated with ablative therapy, follow-up is important to confirm that they have disappeared. Again, if they do not disappear, a biopsy should be performed. If there is any suspicion that a lesion may be more than a wart, a biopsy should be taken before ablation. Rarely, syphilis may present in the secondary phase with condyloma lata (Figure 5.3).

Preoperative investigations

The size of the lesion, the status of the lymph nodes (determined by CT, MRI or PET) and a biopsy should be performed preoperatively. Although imaging may be useful to determine the status of the lymph nodes, no investigation is yet sufficiently reliable to eliminate the need for lymphadenectomy in all but the earliest cases of tumor invasion. A few centers prefer to perform a preoperative sentinel-node assessment using radioactively tagged lymphotropic material (e.g. radiolabeled albumin) injected into the periphery of the primary lesion. This may help with identification of the sentinel node during surgery.

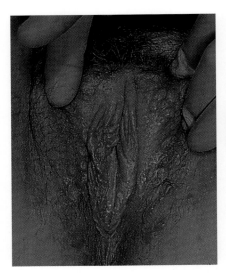

Figure 5.3 Secondary syphilis showing condyloma lata.

Preoperative investigations/management may include:

- full blood count
- urea and electrolytes
- liver function tests
- blood grouping and autologous blood collection or cross-matching
- CT/MRI
- chest X-ray
- ECG
- pelvic examination and Pap smear
- psychosexual counseling
- thromboembolic and antibiotic prophylaxis.

Staging

The staging of vulvar carcinoma has changed greatly over the years. Modern staging is based on surgical rather than clinical findings (Table 5.1). Clinical impression of lymph node status is incorrect in approximately 50% of cases.

Management

VIN is managed by local excision or laser treatment. Imiquimod is another option; one study reported 40% efficacy in multifocal disease,

TABLE 5.1

FIGO staging of vulvar carcinoma

Stage 0	Carcinoma in situ, intraepithelial carcinoma
Stage I	Lesions of $\leq$ 2 cm confined to the vulva or perineum Absence of lymph node metastases
IA	Lesions of $\leq$ 2 cm confined to the vulva or perineum with stromal invasion to a depth of $\leq$ 1 mm No nodal metastases
IB	Lesions of > 2 cm confined to the vulva or perineum with stromal invasion to a depth > 1 mm
Stage II	Vulvar tumor of any size with involvement of the lower third of the urethra, vagina or anus No nodal metastases
Stage III	Tumor of any size on the vulva and/or perineum with:
IIIA(i)	1 lymph node metastasis $\geq$ 5 mm
IIIA(ii)	1–2 lymph node metastases < 5 mm
IIIB(i)	2 or more lymph node metastases $\geq$ 5 mm
IIIB(ii)	3 or more lymph node metastases < 5 mm
Stage IV	
IVA(i)	Tumor invading any of the following: two-thirds upper urethra, bladder mucosa, rectal mucosa or pelvic bone
IVA(ii)	Fixed or ulcerative inguino–femoral nodes
IVB	Any distant metastasis including pelvic lymph nodes

while another reported efficacy of over 80% in women with multifocal and unifocal disease.

The incidence of VIN is increasing. Women with VIN are at high risk for concurrent cervical intraepithelial or vaginal intraepithelial neoplasia (VAIN). It is often found associated with invasive cancer. Excisional surgery is the preferred treatment. Colposcopy is useful but not very accurate. Multiple biopsies are often needed.

Early-stage vulvar tumors with invasion of less than 1 mm may be managed using conservative surgery with a modified partial radical vulvectomy. Essentially, this is a wide local excision with 2-cm margins and a depth as far as possible to the perineal fascia. Recurrences are low and no adjuvant treatment is needed.

In cases of suspected, but unproven, deeper invasion, a two-stage approach (vulvar surgery followed by lymphadenectomy at a later date) may occasionally represent the best option (Figure 5.4). This particularly applies to older patients for whom the extremely mutilating effects of radical vulvectomy and lymphadenectomy are potentially very morbid. The staged approach removes the primary lesion first which can then direct additional therapy including addressing the need for lymph node surgery and or adjuvant radiotherapy. Management should be individualized.

Lesions invasive to a depth of more than 1 mm. The standard management for these lesions is partial radical vulvectomy, again with 2-cm margins. Complete vulvectomy should be considered for rare cases in which disabling adjacent dermatopathology is present. Reconstruction with flaps may be needed to speed recovery.

Radiotherapy can be offered if the surgical margins are less than that considered acceptable, or as primary treatment in young patients with a small primary tumor in the clitoral area. Repeat surgery may be considered if pathological margins are suboptimal.

Lymph node assessment. The lymph nodes are assessed unilaterally in patients with small lateral lesions (e.g. > 2 cm from the midline). Previously, a complete lymphadenectomy was performed for diagnosis and therapy. Currently, vulvar cancer without obvious lymph node metastatic disease appears to be a reasonable indication for sentinel node dissection. Although the radioactive labeling of the sentinel nodes can be scheduled and done before the main operation, it is typically performed at the same time.

Briefly, the lesion is circumferentially injected with radiotracer colloid and an intraoperative handheld detection device is used to find the approximate location of the sentinel node. A lymph node staining dye (e.g. lymph azure) is injected. A small groin incision is made over the previously identified 'hot' area and a dissection carried out to identify

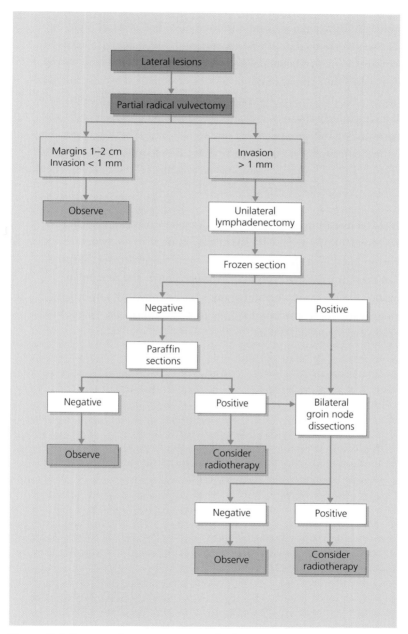

Figure 5.4 Conservative management of vulvar cancer in centers with no access to sentinel node techniques.

blue lymphatic channels and, ideally, a blue 'hot' sentinel node. The sentinel node data are promising but more studies are needed.

Grossly involved inguinal and femoral nodes should be removed if discovered. In addition, midline lesions or unilateral grossly involved nodes indicate the need for surgical bilateral lymph node assessment. If a lymphadenectomy is indicated, it should include the deep nodes surrounding the femoral artery posterior to the cribiform fascia. The lymphadenectomy is usually carried out via separate groin incisions (Figure 5.5). A butterfly incision is now rarely necessary unless the skin bridge over the mons is involved.

Involvement of urethra or anus. Occasionally, women present with involvement of central vital structures. In these cases, neoadjuvant chemotherapy has been proposed to spare the structures. Surgery can then be used with curative intent to remove the remaining lesion. Alternatively, chemotherapy and radiotherapy can be used simultaneously as primary therapy. Again, surgery may be used to remove any residual lesion.

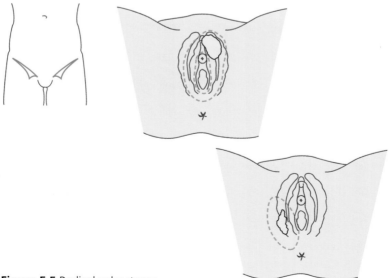

Figure 5.5 Radical vulvectomy.

Where the treatment options are radiotherapy or lymphadenectomy, a randomized trial has indicated that complete lymphadenectomy was therapeutic and superior to adjuvant radiotherapy to the suspected metastatic regional groin nodes.

Postoperative issues

No lymph node involvement. No further treatment may be required after complete radical excision of the tumor if the lymph nodes are not involved. Long-term follow-up by examination, with or without cytology, is still mandatory.

Lymph node involvement. For women with lymph node involvement, external-beam radiotherapy should be given to the groins in case of microscopic metastases. The threshold for recommending adjuvant groin and pelvic radiotherapy varies. It is often recommended if women have one of the following:
- three or more micrometastases (diameter < 5 mm)
- macrometastasis (> 10 mm)
- any presence of extracapsular lymph node spread.

The information obtained from serial microsections and immunohistochemistry of the sentinel node may be sufficient to direct postoperative adjuvant radiotherapy.

Complications. Wound breakdown is the most common postoperative complication, and requires a prolonged hospital stay.

Lymphocyst formation in the groin is another problem, but this may be reduced by using suction drainage. Approximately 5–10% of women will have lymphedema in one or both lower limbs; the use of stockings for the first year postoperatively and prophylactic low-dose antibiotics may be helpful. All of these potentially serious complications may be reduced by the use of sentinel-node techniques.

Prognosis

The prognosis is partly determined by the woman's age. As the initial diagnosis occurs most frequently in women over 70 years of age, age-corrected 5-year survival rates should be quoted. For women with stage I or II disease, the 5-year cancer-related survival rate is over 90% if nodes are not involved. Nodal involvement reduces the rate to approximately 30%, though this depends on the number of nodes involved and whether or not the involvement is bilateral.

Melanoma

Melanoma constitutes the second most common primary vulvar cancer. The prognosis depends on the depth of penetration rather than the diameter of the lesion. Radical local excision is considered for the primary lesion. Sentinel lymph node biopsy has replaced elective lymph node dissection in women with clinically negative nodes. If melanoma is detected, inguinal femoral lymph node dissection is indicated. Interferon α-2b has been used as adjuvant treatment in women with positive nodes. Overall, the prognosis is poor and the survival rate is about 35%.

Primary carcinoma of Bartholin's gland

Primary carcinoma of Bartholin's gland is very rare. Different histological types can occur, including adenocarcinoma, squamous carcinomas, and transitional cell, adenosquamous and adenocystic carcinomas. Delayed diagnosis is common. The lesions are usually deep within the vulva, and extensive deep dissection and inguinofemoral lymphadenectomy is generally required. Postoperative radiotherapy decreases the incidence of local recurrence. Neoadjuvant chemoradiotherapy can reduce the extent of the surgery.

Basal cell carcinoma

Vulvar basal cell carcinomas are rare and occur mostly in postmenopausal white women. The treatment is a wide local excision and approximately 20% local recurrence is reported.

Paget's disease

Paget's disease, seen predominantly in postmenopausal white women, is considered to be an adenocarcinoma in situ. In 10–15% of cases, it is associated with invasive adenocarcinoma (breast, genitourinary, gastrointestinal). The lesions are multifocal and well demarcated, appearing as red eczematous patches. Paget's cells have abundant pale cytoplasm and prominent nuclei arranged in clusters. Wide local excision with 2–5-cm margins is recommended. Different treatment modalities, such as Moh's micrographic surgery, laser ablation, Cavitron ultrasonic aspiration and radiotherapy, have been used. If underlying adenocarcinoma is detected, radical excision and inguinofemoral lymphadenectomy should be performed. The local recurrence rate is high.

Cancer of the urethra

Urethral carcinoma is usually secondary to vulvar carcinoma (stages III and IV). Small lesions are located in the distal half of the urethra, and can be excised with a bilateral inguinofemoral lymphadenectomy. Surgery in conjunction with radiotherapy should be considered for more advanced disease.

Key points – vulvar cancer

- Vulvar intraepithelial neoplasia (VIN) may be treated with local excision or imiquimod.
- Most vulvar cancers are squamous cell carcinomas, which arise from VIN.
- The most common symptom of vulvar cancer is vulvar pruritus.
- The most common physical findings are unifocal vulvar nodule, plaque, ulcer or mass on the labia majora.
- Lymph node dissection is performed for all stages of disease except stage IA.
- More selective wide local radical resection of the primary tumor has replaced radical complete vulvectomy.
- Inguinofemoral lymph node status is the most important predictor of overall prognosis.
- Sentinel node technology is greatly reducing the morbidity associated with groin lymphadenectomy.
- Concurrent chemoradiotherapy has been used in advanced vulvar cancer; however, the role of chemotherapy has not been well studied in this population.

Key references

Judson PL, Habermann EB, Baxter NN, Durham SB, Virnig BA. Trends in the incidence of invasive and in situ vulvar carcinoma. *Obstet Gynecol* 2006;107:1018–22.

Levenback C, Coleman RL, Burke TW, Bodurka-Bevers D, Wolf JK, Gershenson DM. Intraoperative lymphatic mapping and sentinel node identification with blue dye in patients with vulvar cancer. *Gynecol Oncol* 2001;83:276–81.

Gestational trophoblastic neoplasia (GTN) is the term applied to neoplasms resembling the placenta. It describes a spectrum of diseases including hydatidiform mole, invasive mole, choriocarcinoma (Figure 6.1) and placental site tumor.

Until 30–40 years ago, choriocarcinoma had a dismal prognosis. Fortunately, the tumor is chemosensitive, and β-human chorionic gonadotrophin (hCG) is a sensitive and specific tumor marker that allows the identification of women at risk; hCG is an ideal tumor marker as it is able to detect as few as 32 cancer cells. The presence of hCG can indicate the need for aggressive treatment with chemotherapy, surgery and or radiotherapy. Choriocarcinoma is now one of the most curable gynecologic malignancies.

GTN is preceded by a normal pregnancy in 25% of women, and an abortion or ectopic pregnancy in 25%. In 50% of cases, GTN arises spontaneously following fertilization and is in the form of a hydatidiform mole.

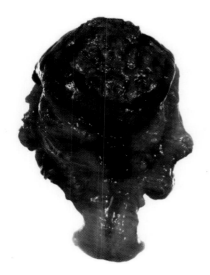

Figure 6.1 Choriocarcinoma arising from uterine body.

GTN can be classified according to the criteria shown in Table 6.1 or with a WHO scoring system (Table 6.2). A FIGO staging system also exists.

Hydatidiform mole

In the UK and USA, hydatidiform mole occurs in 1 in 1200 pregnancies. Its incidence is much higher in the Far East, with reports suggesting it affects 1 in 77 pregnancies in some areas. Maternal age influences the incidence, with lowest rates in the 20–29 years age group, and the highest incidence in mothers under 15 and over 40 years. The incidence does not appear to relate to parity, contraception or irradiation. Paternal factors may also be involved.

TABLE 6.1

Classification of gestational trophoblastic neoplasia

Stage

I   Non-metastatic disease: no evidence of disease outside the uterus

II Metastatic disease: any disease outside the uterus

   A Metastatic disease with a good prognosis

- Short duration (last pregnancy < 4 months)
- Low pretreatment β-hCG titer (< 100 000 IU/24 hours or < 40 000 mIU/mL)
- No metastasis to brain or liver
- No significant previous chemotherapy

   B Metastatic disease with a poor prognosis

- Long duration (last pregnancy > 4 months)
- High pretreatment β-hCG titer (> 100 000 IU/24 hours or > 40 000 mIU/mL)
- Brain or liver metastasis
- Significant previous chemotherapy
- Term pregnancy

Adapted from Hammond et al. *Am J Obstet Gynecol* 1973;115:451–7.
hCG, human chorionic gonadotrophin.

TABLE 6.2

WHO scoring system for gestational trophoblastic neoplasia based on prognostic factors

Prognostic factor	Score*			
	0	1	2	4
Age (years)	< 40	≥ 40	–	–
Antecedent pregnancy	Mole	Abortion	Term	–
Interval†	< 4	≥ 4 but < 7	≥ 7 but < 13	≥ 13
Pretreatment serum β-hCG (IU/mL)	< 1000	1000 to < 10 000	10 000 to < 100 000	≥ 100 000
Largest tumor, including uterine tumor	–	3 to < 5 cm	≥ 5 cm	–
Site of metastases	Lung	Spleen, kidney	Gastrointestinal tract	Brain, liver
Number of metastases identified	–	1–4	5–8	> 8
Prior failed chemotherapy drugs	–	–	Single drug	2 or more

*The total score for a woman is obtained by adding the individual scores for each prognostic factor. Total score < 6 = low risk; score ≥ 7 = high risk.
†Interval time (months) between end of antecedent pregnancy and start of chemotherapy.
FIGO staging for gestational trophoblastic neoplasia 2000. *Int J Gynecol Obstet* 2002; 77:285.
hCG, human chorionic gonadotropin.

Hydatidiform mole can be either complete or partial. In complete moles, no fetus is present and the placenta is composed entirely of vesicular tissue. An 'empty' oocyte is fertilized and the male haploid DNA set duplicates to create a diploid karyotype, 46XX. Occasionally, two sperm, one carrying 23X and the other 23Y jointly fertilize the empty oocyte giving the diploid 46XY. In a partial mole, the fetus usually dies in the first or second trimester, and so there is fetal tissue, often with a triploid karyotype. Differences between the two types are summarized in Table 6.3.

Postmolar GTN. The risk of developing GTN from a mole is related to certain risk factors, the most important of which is diagnosis of a complete mole. Women with a recently diagnosed complete mole and all three of the following risk factors have a two-fold increase in risk of developing a rising hCG level after evacuation of the uterus:

- very high β-hCG levels (i.e. > 100 000 IU/mL)
- prolonged vaginal bleeding
- large thecal luteal cyst.

Approximately 30% of women with all three risk factors will require chemotherapy some time in the future. This high probability may justify prophylactic chemotherapy. Also known as a chemotherapy 'umbrella', women with a complete mole who are unlikely to comply with weekly

TABLE 6.3

Differences between complete and partial hydatidiform moles

Complete moles	Partial moles
• Most common form	• Account for 10–15%
• No fetal tissue present	• Some fetal tissue present
• Normal karyotype (usually 46XX)	
• Localized gestational trophoblastic neoplasia develops in 15% of evacuated complete moles	• Less likely to progress
• Choriocarcinoma develops in 4% of evacuated complete moles	
• More likely to require chemotherapy (7–12% of cases)	• Less likely to require chemotherapy (3% of cases)

hCG testing can be offered chemotherapy immediately before the evacuation. This can reduce the risk of postmolar GTN to close to zero.

Diagnosis

Women usually present with delayed menses, signs of pregnancy, vaginal bleeding or passage of vesicular tissue vaginally. In addition, the risk of developing pre-eclampsia and hyperthyroidism is greatly increased. However, most women in the developed world are asymptomatic at diagnosis and this is partly a reflection of the high utilization of ultrasound in nearly all pregnancies. The diagnosis is strongly suggested by ultrasound and many moles are now picked up on routine antenatal scans.

Partial hydatidiform mole may be diagnosed on ultrasound, but it is often only detected when aborted material is examined histologically. This is because a fetus is seen on ultrasound and the presumed diagnosis is missed abortion. If measured, β-hCG will be elevated, but this can also occur in normal pregnancy.

Management

Investigations for women with GTN include:
- full history and examination
- chest X-ray
- pretreatment serum β-hCG
- full blood count
- urea, electrolytes, thyroid-stimulating hormone (TSH), and liver function tests.

If any of these are abnormal, CT of the brain, chest, abdomen and pelvis should be performed.

Evacuation. If the diagnosis has been established, evacuation should be performed with suction curettage. For women with a grossly enlarged uterus, laparotomy facilities should be available, though a hysterotomy or hysterectomy is rarely required. Follow-up after evacuation should follow the plan shown in Table 6.4.

The actual evacuation is similar to a common elective pregnancy termination or evacuation for a missed abortion, though there is an increased amount of bleeding. This can be reduced by using continuous

TABLE 6.4

Post-evacuation follow-up of hydatidiform moles

- Measurement of β-hCG levels every 1–2 weeks until negative on two occasions, then bimonthly for 1 year. Contraception should be used for 6–12 months; the combined oral contraceptive pill is not contraindicated
- Physical examination including pelvic examination every 2 weeks until remission, then every 3 months for 1 year
- Initial chest film; repeat only if the β-hCG titer plateaus or rises
- Chemotherapy started immediately if:
  - the β-hCG titer rises or plateaus during follow-up
  - metastases are detected at any time

hCG, human chorionic gonadotropin.
Modified from DiSaia and Creasman. *Clinical Gynecologic Oncology*, 4th edn.
St Louis: Mosby, 1993.

ultrasound guidance and starting oxytocin as soon as the suction device is inserted into the uterus. If tumor is noted on the vagina, a biopsy should not be taken because doing so will lead to bleeding.

A repeat evacuation is sometimes performed when women are referred to a specialist. If a prolonged interval has occurred between the initial diagnosis of postmolar GTN and planned chemotherapy, a large amount of uterine disease and bleeding may have developed. Although the risk of perforation is real, repeat evacuation with ultrasound guidance of a cavity filled with recurrent disease can be considered. Ideally, women should begin chemotherapy immediately and not require a second evacuation.

Metastasis. Chemotherapy is the preferred treatment for all metastatic disease. Rarely, surgery may be considered for an isolated persistent chemoresistant metastasis.

Recurrence

Prediction. There are several systems that predict risk of recurrence of GTN. These can be used to identify those patients who need chemotherapy and the regimen that should be used. Various modifications have been reported; the original Charing Cross system (non-metastatic/metastatic with good or poor prognosis) is simple yet achieves high cure rates with reasonable triage of women into single or multi-agent regimens.

Chemotherapy. The indications for chemotherapy are:
- a diagnosis of choriocarcinoma
- a rise or plateau of β-hCG levels
- imaging indicating new metastatic disease.

Typically, with appropriate monitoring (i.e. weekly serum β-hCG levels), the first indication for chemotherapy will be a rise in β-hCG level. Because the assay has a coefficient of variation of approximately 10%, a rise must be shown from samples taken on days 1, 7 and 14 before a true rise can be claimed. Another β-hCG pattern occasionally used to indicate a need for chemotherapy is a prolonged (e.g. > 12 weeks) slow fall in β-hCG level.

Selecting a regimen. Any validated scoring system can be applied to determine the need for single agent or multi-agent chemotherapy once chemotherapy is indicated. Women with a high-risk score (e.g. WHO > 8) are prescribed multi-agent regimens because of the increased risk of failure with single-agent regimens. Single-agent chemotherapy is an appropriate option for women at low risk (e.g. WHO < 4).

Methotrexate and actinomycin are the usual drugs used in single-agent regimens. There are no clear advantages of one over the other. Actinomycin can be administered every 14 days, but it is a strong vesicant. Methotrexate, available in an oral formulation, has a relatively wide therapeutic window so it is easier to administer in low resource settings. Other active drugs include oral 5-fluorouracil analogs and platinum agents.

After a single-agent regimen has failed, switching to the other available single-agent drug is usually recommended. Once this second agent fails to have any effect, or if the woman has a high-risk score, multi-agent therapy is usually tried.

Choriocarcinoma is treated with multi-agent regimens whenever it is diagnosed. A commonly used regimen includes etoposide, methothrexate, actinomycin, cyclophosphamide and vincristine (EMA-CO). Other, less complicated, platinum-containing regimens are also available. None has a clear advantage.

Placental site trophoblastic tumor

Placental site trophoblastic tumor, a rare entity, comprises intermediate trophoblast. Human placental lactogen is a marker of disease progression and recurrence. The β-hCG is usually low. Treatment is surgical hysterectomy because the tumor is insensitive to chemotherapy.

False-positive β-hCG

ACOG reports that some women have factors circulating in their serum that interact with the β-hCG antibody, causing false-positive results. Methods of checking the result include:

- urine pregnancy test
- repeat assay with serial dilutions of serum
- pre-absorbing serum
- using a different assay.

Caution should be exercised whenever clinical findings and laboratory results are discordant.

Quiescent gestational trophoblastic disease

Quiescent gestational trophoblastic disease is characterized by a persistently low level of β-hCG after a molar pregnancy. It is considered to result from the presence of highly differentiated non-invasive syncytiotrophoblast cells. It is reported that 6–10% of women with quiescent gestational trophoblastic disease will eventually develop overt disease that requires therapy. The presence of hyperglycosylated β-hCG indicates invasive rather than quiescent disease (a specific assay is available).

Prognosis

With modern chemotherapy, most women with GTN can be cured (Table 6.5), retaining their uterus and fertility. Even when recurrence occurs, the results achieved with further treatment can be impressive. The indications for hysterectomy include uncontrollable bleeding and a single residual focus of disease.

TABLE 6.5

Survival by FIGO stage in women with gestational trophoblastic disease treated in 1996–1998

Stage	Number of women (n = 459)	Overall survival (%)		
		1 year	2 years	5 years
I	358	99.7	99.4	99.4
II	23	95.6	86.2	86.2
III	59	89.7	89.7	87.6
IV	19	78.4	72.6	72.6

FIGO, International Federation of Gynecology and Obstetrics.
Data from Ngan HY et al. *Int J Gynaecol Obstet* 2003;83:167.

Key points – gestational trophoblastic neoplasia

- Serum β-human chorionic gonadotrophin (hCG) level should be checked in a woman with persistent unexplained bleeding.
- Gestational trophoblastic neoplasia (GTN) includes hydatidiform mole, invasive mole, choriocarcinoma and placental-site tumor.
- Surgical evacuation is the first-line treatment of molar disease.
- With modern chemotherapy, most women with GTN can be cured, retaining their uterus and fertility.
- Use of an effective contraception is encouraged during the full interval of hCG follow-up.
- Single-agent chemotherapy is recommended for women with stage I disease who want to retain fertility.
- Etoposide, methotrexate, actinomycin D, cyclophosphamide, vincristine (EMA-CO) is the recommended chemotherapy for women with metastasis and high-risk prognostic scores.

Key references

Hammond CB, Borchet LG, Tyrey L et al. Treatment of metastatic trophoblastic disease: good and poor prognosis. *Am J Obstet Gynecol* 1973;115:451–7.

Ngan S, Seckl MJ. Gestational trophoblastic neoplasia management: an update. *Curr Opin Oncol* 2007;19:486–91.

Sebire NJ, Seckl MJ. Gestational trophoblastic disease: current management of hydatidiform mole. *BMJ* 2008;337:a1193(doi: 10.1136/bmj.a1193).

Pain is considered to be a complex experience embracing physical, mental, social and behavioral processes, and compromising the quality of life of many individuals. Prompt and effective management of pain is achievable for most women. For those with pain resistant to initial treatment, perseverance and referral to a specialist at a chronic pain center is necessary.

Pain may be broadly divided into two distinct groups:

- nociceptive, which occurs where there is tissue damage
- neuropathic, which results from damage to, or an abnormality in, the nervous system.

Cancer-associated pain

Cancer and pain are inextricably linked in the minds of individuals and, unfortunately, many doctors. Pain associated with cancer may be caused by the erosive effects of the tumor itself or by treatment (e.g. radiation plexopathy and constipation secondary to opioid administration). It may also result from muscle spasm or musculoskeletal problems arising from the consequences of the illness. A woman may, therefore, complain of various different types of pain.

Tumor erosion, muscle spasm and bony secondaries will produce nociceptive pain, which may be sharp and stabbing, cramping or throbbing. Neuropathic pain produced by damage to the nervous tissue is characteristically shooting, lancinating, burning or described as feeling like electric shocks. It is often associated with paresthesias and dysesthesias.

Severity of pain may increase in proportion to either tumor mass or the occurrence of new metastases. A tumor enlarging within a fibrous capsule causes continuous pain, which is gradual in onset, tending to start with an ache. Those involving a hollow viscus, such as the small intestine, interfere with peristaltic function and cause cramp-like or colicky abdominal pain. Tumors may become inflamed or infected, which will also produce pain; subsequent necrosis causes tenderness and pain.

Tumors can invade bone through direct invasion or distant metastasis. Vulvar and cervical carcinomas invade bone directly, while other tumors usually spread to bone by distant metastasis. Most gynecologic tumors, however, do not usually metastasize to bone.

Nerve involvement. Tumors characteristically cause shooting or stabbing pain, radiating along the path of the nerve. This happens as a result of direct infiltration and also from stretching or compressing nerves, particularly where the nerve lies against bone or within a bony cavity. For example, the lumbar and sacral plexuses may be infiltrated by primary and metastatic tumors in the pelvis, causing severe pain in the lower part of the back, pelvis and lower limbs. If the lower sacral plexus is involved, severe pain may be experienced in the perineum.

Isolated peripheral nerves, or their roots, may be affected by tumors in the pelvis. Involvement of the sciatic nerve, for instance, may produce pain radiating down the back of the leg into the foot. The lumbosacral plexuses may also be damaged by radiotherapy, producing radiation neuritis or plexopathy, which may present with pain or sensory/motor deficits. Pain caused by nerve involvement may be associated with sensory abnormalities such as dysesthesias or paresthesias. Women may complain of, or present with, motor or sensory deficits as well as pain.

Infiltration of the vascular system. Direct infiltration of arteries, veins and lymphatics occurs with gynecologic cancer because of the close anatomic relationship in the pelvis. Arterial and venous involvement causes ischemic pain and venous engorgement, respectively, distal to the blockage. Lymphatic involvement produces the distressing problem of lymphedema distal to the blockage. Lymphedema may be particularly painful and can easily be overlooked. Lymphedematous legs are heavy to move and may cause pain by traction on intrapelvic structures.

Pain relief
Curative cancer treatment, using surgery, radiotherapy or chemotherapy, usually provides relief from pain being caused directly by the tumor. Even when such measures are not curative, they may be invaluable for the palliation of pain not easily controlled by standard measures.

Indeed, radiotherapy is the treatment of choice for some women, such as those with isolated bone secondaries.

Effective postoperative analgesia is particularly important following oncological surgery, as persisting pain is associated, in the minds of patients, with persisting cancer. Many centers now have the option of epidural anesthesia in the perioperative period following major gynecologic surgery. Patient-controlled and continuous intravenous administration of opioid drugs has also improved the quality of postoperative analgesia.

Prospective surveys suggest 70–90% of people with cancer could have cancer-related pain adequately relieved by systemic administration of drug therapies. Fear of addiction or fear of tolerance can be barriers to effective pain management. Pain screening and assessment should be performed systematically using pain assessment scores to define the severity of discomfort (see *Fast Facts: Chronic Pain*).

Analgesic drugs can be divided into non-opioid, opioid and adjuvant or non-conventional analgesic drugs.

General principles. Analgesics should be prescribed for pain, with the dose titrated to the woman's response. There is no merit in giving an inadequate dose (as assessed on body weight) infrequently with the aim of avoiding 'addiction'. There is no evidence that using opioids at a dose high enough to relieve pain carries any appreciable risk of addiction. It is unlikely that a woman with pain resulting from gynecologic malignancy (with or without metastatic disease) who has not had a curative operation will be effectively treated without recourse to opioids, alone or in combination. The use of opioid analgesic medication should not be seen as a last resort, nor should it be reserved until pain is intolerable. Early and effective analgesia improves the quality of patients' lives and may possibly improve longevity. The WHO has produced a three-step analgesic ladder for cancer pain control (Figure 7.1).

Pain in patients with malignancy may not be due to the underlying disease. Up to 30% of patients presenting with a diagnosis of cancer have been found to have pain unrelated to the underlying condition. The pain results from treatment in approximately 5% of cases, concurrent

119

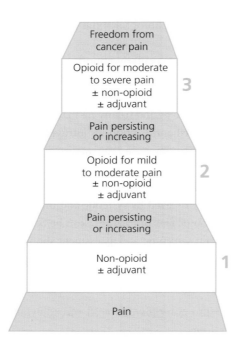

Figure 7.1 WHO analgesic stairway. Reproduced with permission from WHO.

disorders such as osteoarthritis or migraine in 22%, and relates to debilities such as bedsores in 6% of patients. Pain diaries kept by patients and the use of visual analog pain scores may help in the provision of effective analgesia.

Non-opioid analgesics include paracetamol (acetaminophen), aspirin and non-steroidal anti-inflammatory drugs (NSAIDs) (Table 7.1). Paracetamol is a good minor analgesic that does not cause gastrointestinal problems but does not have an anti-inflammatory action; hepatotoxicity is a potential side effect. Acetylsalicylic acid (ASA; aspirin) has anti-inflammatory properties and may be helpful for treating non-visceral pain. NSAIDs such as indometacin, diclofenac and ketorolac can provide stronger analgesia with anti-inflammatory effects. All the NSAIDs cause gastrointestinal irritation, which may lead to gastric ulceration and hemorrhage. There is no convincing evidence that the route of administration of NSAID alters the incidence of gastrointestinal side effects. NSAIDs may reduce renal function, which, in some individuals, can lead to renal failure; this occurs more

TABLE 7.1

Doses and routes of some non-opioid analgesics

Dose	Interval (hours)	Route	Maximum daily dose	Comments
Paracetamol (acetaminophen)				
500–1000 mg	4–6	Oral/rectal	Oral, 4000 mg; 3600 mg	Liquid available
Aspirin				
500–1000 mg	4–6	Oral/rectal	4000 mg	
Diflunisal				
500 mg	8	Oral	1500 mg	First dose 1000 mg
Choline magnesium trisalicylate (not licensed in the UK)				
750–1500 mg	8–12	Oral	3000 mg	Liquid available; less dyspepsia and platelet dysfunction
Ibuprofen				
200–600 mg	4–6	Oral	2400 mg	
Ketoprofen				
25–75 mg	4–8	Oral	300 mg	
Flurbiprofen				
50–100 mg	4–6	Oral	300 mg	
Naproxen				
250 mg	6–8	Oral	1250 mg	Sustained release available; first dose 500 mg

CONTINUED

TABLE 7.1 (CONTINUED)

Indometacin

25–50 mg	8–12	Oral/rectal	100 mg	Frequent side effects

Ketorolac

10–30 mg	6	Oral	40 mg	Lower dose for repeated use
		i.v./i.m.	60 mg	Limit to 5 days (orally/i.v.)

Etodolac

200–400 mg	6–8	Oral	1200 mg	

i.m., intramuscular; i.v. intravenous.

commonly in the elderly. There may also be exacerbation of reversible airways obstruction in susceptible individuals. Despite these side effects, this class of drug may be very effective, particularly in the treatment of bony metastases.

Opioids. When non-opioid drugs fail to provide effective pain relief, as is often the case with moderate and severe pain, opioid analgesia should be started (Table 7.2). Women should be started on weaker agents but if these fail to give satisfactory relief, attending physicians should have no hesitation in promptly switching to appropriate doses of stronger opioids. Evaluation of opioid responsiveness is based on individualization of the dose. This is critical to successful opioid treatment; there is no 'one' correct dose. The endpoint is adequate pain relief or intolerable and unmanageable side effects.

Dose increments are 25% to 150%, depending on the circumstances. The responsiveness of an individual patient to a specific drug cannot be determined unless the dose reaches treatment-limiting toxicity. Treatment side effects may limit responsiveness and therefore should be addressed as an essential element of effective opioid therapy.

TABLE 7.2

Equivalent opioid doses

Drug	Oral dose	Parenteral dose
Morphine sulfate, parenteral		10 mg every 4 hours
Morphine sulfate, oral	30 mg, every 4 hours	
Morphine sulfate, controlled release	90 mg every 12 hours	Not available
Codeine	200 mg every 4 hours	100–120 mg every 4 hours
Oxycodone	15–20 mg every 4 hours	Not available
Oxycodone, controlled release	45–60 mg every 12 hours	Not available
Hydromorphone	8 mg every 4 hours	1.5–3.0 mg every 4 hours
Levorphanol	4 mg every 6–8 hours	2 mg every 6–8 hours
Meperidine	300 mg every 2–3 hours	100 mg every 2–3 hours
Methadone	20 mg* every 6–12 hours	10 mg every 6 hours

*A dose ratio of 1:4 (1 mg of oral methadone = 4 mg of oral morphine) is used for patients receiving less than 90 mg of morphine. Patients receiving 90–300 mg/day receive methadone at a ratio of 1:8. Finally, a ratio of 1:12 is used for patients receiving morphine doses above 300 mg/day.

For intermediate pain not relieved by NSAIDs, codeine, 30–60 mg every 4 hours, or dihydrocodeine, 30 mg every 4–6 hours, can be used. These drugs, which tend to cause constipation, should be taken after food.

If codeine or dihydrocodeine fail to relieve pain, an opioid with a short half-life, used on an 'as needed' basis, can be tried. For constant pain, a sustained-release preparation (available orally for morphine and oxycodone and transdermally for fentanyl) can be used. Methadone and levorphanol have long half-lives (22 and 16 hours, respectively). Both are efficiently absorbed by the gut and both methadone and levorphanol can be taken rectally, sublingually and parenterally. Methadone is effective in controlling neuropathic pain and preventing opioid tolerance; it causes specific antagonism of the N-methyl D-aspartate receptors in the dorsal horn of the spinal cord.

Tramadol hydrochloride is a synthetic analog of codeine that inhibits norepinephrine (noradrenaline) and serotonin uptake. It is used extensively in countries where there are restrictions on opioid prescription and it may be of value in the treatment of cancer pain in patients resistant to using morphine or similar drugs. It can cause seizures at high doses, and it is expensive.

If patients are in severe pain, the daily dose of morphine required may be determined by allowing the patient to self-medicate using oral morphine linctus taken hourly as required or delivered by patient-controlled intravenous infusion. The amount of morphine used over 24 hours can be calculated and an initial daily or twice-daily dose determined. Alternatively, when the patient is not in hospital, the dose can be increased from an estimated starting point until pain is relieved. Doses for breakthrough pain should always be prescribed and patients should never be unable to self-medicate in the event of an increase in pain.

Patient-controlled analgesia (PCA) is helpful for initiation of parenteral opioid therapy. PCA will indicate the 24-hour opioid requirement, allowing the non-parenteral dose of opioid to be estimated.

The mu receptors mediating systemic morphine analgesia differ from those responsible for respiratory depression and constipation. Fentanyl analgesia receptors differ from those responsible for morphine analgesia. The side effects of opioid therapy are commonly constipation and somnolence. Less common side effects include nausea, myoclonus, itch, headache, sweating, amenorrhea, sexual dysfunction and urinary retention.

When there is a poor response to opioids:
- lower the opioid requirement by using the spinal route of administration or by adding non-opioid or adjuvant analgesia

- improve the management of side effects
- examine non-pharmacological means of lowering the opioid requirement.

Patients receiving strong painkillers will often need some time to determine the drug dose that adequately controls their pain. When this dose has been established, they may be controlled on a stable-dose regimen with regular review. Increasing dose requirements do not necessarily mean that tolerance to opioid drugs has developed. It may indicate progression of established disease or the development of new disease.

Antidepressant drugs are used widely in the management of chronic pain. They are the only drugs of proven value in the treatment of post-herpetic neuralgia and may well be useful in patients with neuropathic pain due to malignancy or its treatment (Table 7.3). The older tricyclic agents may be more effective in this role than the selective serotonin reuptake inhibitors, such as fluoxetine or paroxetine. Exactly how antidepressants work in the treatment of pain is not fully understood. Modulation of descending cortical inhibitory pathways, positive effects on mood, and changes in central spinal processing have been suggested as modes of action.

Anticonvulsant and membrane-stabilizing agents. Anticonvulsant drugs such as carbamazepine and membrane-stabilizing agents such as lidocaine and mexiletine (not in the UK) may be of benefit in alleviating neuropathic pain (Table 7.3).

Intravenous steroids may be tried when pain is due to swelling of the tumor. They may be of particular benefit for intracranial metastases and spinal cord compression. Intravenous dexamethasone, 4–10 mg every 4–6 hours, appears to be the drug of choice.

Pain resulting from radiotherapy. Radiation may cause tissue fibrosis involving the sacral and lumbar plexuses, causing sensory and motor deficits and neuropathic pain. The pain may be exacerbated by movements that stretch or produce tension in the nerve roots. Skin reactions occur during radiotherapy causing burning pain, which can be alleviated using 0.1% hydrocortisone cream or topical local anesthetic creams.

TABLE 7.3

Some adjuvant analgesic drugs used to relieve pain associated with cancer

Class	Drug	Approximate daily dosage	Route
Tricyclic anti-depressants	Amitriptyline hydrochloride	10–150 mg	Oral/i.m.
	Clomipramine hydrochloride	10–150 mg	Oral
	Desipramine hydrochloride	10–150 mg	Oral
	Doxepin	12.5–150 mg	Oral/i.m.
	Imipramine hydrochloride	12.5–150 mg	Oral
SSRIs	Fluoxetine	20–60 mg	Oral
	Paroxetine	10–40 mg	Oral
Anti-convulsants	Carbamazepine	100–1200 mg	Oral
	Clonazepam	2–10 mg	Oral
	Gabapentin	300 mg–3.6 g	Oral
Membrane stabilizers	Mexiletine	150–1000 mg	Oral

i.m., intramuscular; SSRI, selective serotonin reuptake inhibitor.

Pain resulting from chemotherapy. Chemotherapy can cause pain from direct cytotoxic activity and from the production of peripheral neuropathy. For example, vincristine can cause tingling and numbness in the fingers and toes. The pain from peripheral neuropathies often decreases with time, but it may be quite disabling and refractory to treatment. Antidepressants may be of great benefit.

Both vincristine and vinblastine can cause myalgia and arthralgia, while procarbazine and 5-fluorouracil can cause neurotoxicity. All cytotoxics can cause mucosal reactions in the gastrointestinal tract – symptoms relate to the lips, mouth, pharynx, stomach and colon. Mucositis may be intensely painful and difficult to treat. Local anesthetics, such as lozenges, linctus or aerosols, can be helpful.

Alternative therapies. Transcutaneous electrical nerve stimulation (TENS), acupuncture, aromatherapy, hypnotherapy and psychological therapies can all be helpful in the management of malignant pain.

Interventional pain management techniques. When conservative management techniques fail, more invasive techniques should be considered. These might include nerve blocks, epidural/intrathecal administration of drugs and neurodestructive procedures. An algorithm for the management of continuing pain in patients with cancer is shown in Figure 7.2.

Gastrointestinal symptoms

Obstruction. Hollow organs can be invaded by gynecologic tumors. If the bowel is involved, a cramping colicky pain may result. Bowel obstruction can be relieved by surgical resection of the involved segment; patients may require a colostomy and, if this is the case, will benefit from preoperative counseling. High end-stage obstruction may require a percutaneous gastrostomy. Stents may also help. Bowel hypomobility may be temporary and related to the surgery; it can also be a manifestation of disseminated intraperitoneal cancer or it may be associated with a paraneoplastic phenomenon.

Hyoscine hydrobromide may be helpful for women with bowel obstruction, as it acts on the vomiting center and decreases gastrointestinal secretions and intestinal tone. In women for whom surgery is unsuitable, conservative management of obstruction at high or low levels may require a trial of corticosteroids, which work mostly by decreasing the inflammatory edema. The conservative medical approach to high bowel obstruction has improved the palliative approach for women near to death.

Constipation and diarrhea are also common problems. Constipation often results from oral opioid therapy, so women receiving opioid analgesia regularly should also be given laxatives. Fecal impaction is a potent cause of severe rectal pain. Good hydration, adequate levels of dietary fiber and the use of other bulking or hydrophilic agents are, therefore, essential. If laxatives are needed, either a stimulant laxative such as bisacodyl, 5–10 mg at night, or senna granules, 5–10 mL at night, are useful. If these are unsuccessful, osmotic agents such as glycerine suppositories and, in extreme cases, olive oil enemas and manual evacuation may be required. Mu receptor

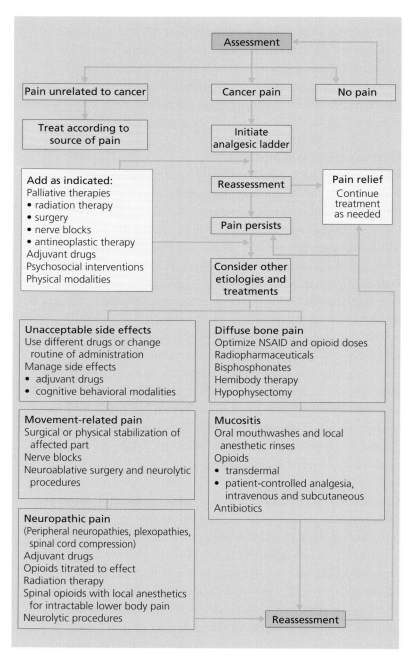

Figure 7.2 Managing continual pain in patients with cancer.

antagonists, e.g. methylnaltrexone, are effective in relieving opioid constipation.

Diarrhea in progressive gynecologic cancer can be a sign of fecal impaction. After excluding the possibility of *Clostridium difficile* infection, diphenoxylate and atropine (4 tablets initially, then 2 tablets 6-hourly until relief occurs) or loperamide (4 mg initially, then 2 mg after each loose bowel motion until relief occurs) can be considered. If these are ineffective, codeine phosphate, 30 mg orally three or four times a day, or 15, 30 or 60 mg intramuscularly, can be used. Anticholinergic derivatives, corticosteroids and opioids can be used for women with diarrhea and tenesmus.

If rectovaginal or enterovaginal fistula is present, surgical repair or diversion should be considered. If surgery is not feasible, the area should be kept clean; octreotide can be used to reduce the drainage from a small bowel fistula.

Dry mouth/oropharynx. During cancer or its treatment, the mouth and oropharynx can become dry, causing much discomfort. This can be relieved by mouthwashes, sucking on ice cubes or acid sweets, or by chewing gum. It is also important to counter dehydration and prevent infection. Maintaining good oral and dental hygiene can do much to prevent infection. Prompt treatment of oral candidiasis with nystatin lozenges or suspension is helpful.

Hiccups are a gastrointestinal side effect that can cause much distress; they may be relieved by inhaling carbon dioxide (i.e. by breathing into a paper bag). If this fails, a phenothiazine such as chlorpromazine hydrochloride, 25 mg orally three times daily, is usually effective. Alternatively, dexamfetamine sulphate (amfetamine sulfate), 2.5–5 mg three times daily, or hyoscine, at a starting dose of 300 mg, which is repeated 2 hours later, can be used.

Nausea and vomiting may be caused directly by the tumor, by chemotherapy and radiotherapy or by opioid medication.

Three distinct types of chemotherapy-induced emesis have been reported:

- acute emesis, occurring within 1–2 hours of chemotherapy

- delayed emesis, appearing during the day following chemotherapy
- anticipatory emesis, occurring before treatment.

A classification scheme has been established to reflect the likelihood of emesis following treatment with different chemotherapeutic agents (Table 7.4).

The three categories of drugs used to counter emesis are corticosteroids, type three 5-hydroxytryptamine ($5HT_3$) receptor antagonists and the neurokinin-1 receptor antagonist aprepitant. Women receiving high-risk emetogenic regimens benefit from a combination of aprepitant with $5HT_3$ antagonists and corticosteroids. Those experiencing delayed emesis require maintenance therapy with a combination of aprepitant and dexamethasone. Women receiving moderate-risk emetogenic regimens require a $5HT_3$ antagonist plus dexamethasone. Dexamethasone or a $5HT_3$ antagonist alone can prevent delayed emesis in this population. Women receiving low-risk emetogenic regimens require dexamethasone, 8 mg, as a single agent. Behavioral therapy or benzodiazepines have been suggested to help patients who develop anticipatory emesis.

Nausea in terminally ill cancer patients can be caused by the drugs used, autonomic failure, peptic ulcer disease, constipation, bowel obstruction, metabolic abnormalities and increased intracranial pressure. All of these causes should be managed aggressively. Prokinetic agents, such as metoclopramide, are often helpful because of the combination of central and gastric-emptying effects. Haloperidol, octreotide, hyoscine and finally midazolam, for palliative sedation, can be used.

Urinary tract problems

Involvement of the urinary tract causes pain in the loin and groin that may range from a dull ache to colic. Cervical tumors often cause hydronephrosis and fistula formation. Ureteric blockage may be relieved by either removing the compressing tumor or using ureteric stents. Nephrostomy tubes can be used if it is impossible to pass either antegrade or retrograde ureteric stents. These techniques are also useful for patients who require palliative urinary diversion as a result of cancer causing urinary fistulas. Occasionally tumors can cause urethral

TABLE 7.4

Emetogenicity of chemotherapy drugs

Emetic risk (incidence of emesis without antiemetics)	Chemotherapy drug
High (> 90%)	Cisplatin
	Mechlorethamine
	Streptozotocin
	Cyclophosphamide $\geq$ 1500 mg/m^2
	Carmustine
	Dacarbazine
	Dactinomycin
Moderate (30–90%)	Oxaliplatin
	Cytarabine > 1 g/m^2
	Carboplatin
	Ifosfamide
	Cyclophosphamide < 1500 mg/m^2
	Doxorubicin
	Daunorubicin
	Epirubicin
	Idarubicin
	Irinotecan
Low (10–30%)	Paclitaxel
	Docetaxel
	Mitoxantrone
	Topotecan
	Etoposide
	Pemetrexed
	Methotrexate
	Mitomycin
	Gemcitabine
	Cytarabine $\leq$ 1000 mg/m^2
	Fluorouracil
	Bortezomib
	Cetuximab
	Trastuzumab

CONTINUED

TABLE 7.4 (CONTINUED)	
Minimal (< 10%)	Bevacizumab
	Bleomycin
	Busulfan
	2-Chlorodeoxyadenosine
	Fludarabine
	Rituximab
	Vinblastine
	Vincristine
	Vinorelbine

Modified from Kris et al. *J Clin Oncol* 2006;24:2932–47.

obstruction resulting in complete retention; this must be relieved by catheterization. Prompt recognition and treatment of urinary tract infection is also important for relieving associated pain and preventing ascending infection, with its associated risk of pyelonephritis.

Psychological problems

Depression and anxiety affect 10–15% of cancer patients. In addition to depressed mood, dysphoria, loss of energy and hopelessness, it may present as an increase in the level of pain expression or dissocial behavior. Antidepressants and serotonin reuptake inhibitors are useful. Women with major depression should be referred to a psychiatrist.

Delirium is diagnosed based on an alteration in the patient's cognition, impairment of consciousness and neuropsychiatric symptoms. It can be a side effect of opioid treatment. Differential diagnoses are dementia and depression. Haloperidol is used to treat the symptoms, but the underlying causes of delirium should also be addressed.

Dyspnea

Shortness of breath should be assessed during rest and exertion. Treatment is guided by the underlying process, which should be investigated on a case-by-case basis. If severe malignant pleural effusion is detected, pleurodesis or an indwelling pleural catheter is recommended. An indwelling pleural catheter can be considered for debilitated patients with a short life expectancy who opt for outpatient treatment, and for those in whom pleurodesis cannot be performed.

Anorexia

Catabolic syndrome is the manifestation of paraneoplastic anorexia/cachexia. Extreme weight loss can be related to starvation. Megestrol acetate and medroxyprogesterone, corticosteroids, prokinetic agents and nutritional support can be beneficial.

Lymphedema

Lymphedema is a troublesome condition in patients with cancer and occurs in 5–10% of women with vulvar cancer. It also presents occasionally in women after the treatment of cervical and endometrial neoplasia.

Lymphedema should be treated by elevation and the use of graduated compression bandages. Low-dose antibiotics should be used prophylactically in women suffering from intermittent infection of edematous legs; the infections are usually staphylococcal or streptococcal.

For women with more troublesome symptoms, intermittent positive pressure boots can be used for 1–2 hours during the day to reduce the volume of lymph. Lymphedema should be distinguished from deep venous thrombosis.

Bleeding

The risk of bleeding from a progressive tumor should be explained to the woman and her family. Emergency palliative sedation with midazolam or lorazepam can be considered. Palliative radiotherapy can be used in some cases. Acute bleeding should be managed on a case-by-case basis.

Key points – pain management and palliation

- Pain is considered to be a complex experience embracing physical, mental, social and behavioral processes.
- Ask the woman: "What do you feel is wrong." Do not presume to second guess her.
- Prompt effective management of pain is achievable for most women.
- Women receiving strong painkillers will often need some time to determine the drug dose that adequately controls their pain.
- Nausea and vomiting may be caused directly by the tumor, by chemotherapy and radiotherapy or by opioid medication.
- Most symptoms can be treated.
- Depression and anxiety affect 10–15% of cancer patients.

Key references

American Society of Clinical Oncology, Kris MG, Hesketh PJ, Somerfield MR et al. American Society of Clinical Oncology guideline for antiemetics in oncology: update 2006. *J Clin Oncol* 2006;24:2932–47. Erratum in: *J Clin Oncol* 2006;24:5341–2.

Cepeda MS, Cousins MJ, Carr DB. *Fast Facts: Chronic Pain*. Oxford: Health Press Ltd, 2007.

Clayton JM, Butow PN, Tattersall MH et al. Randomized controlled trial of a prompt list to help advanced cancer patients and their caregivers to ask questions about prognosis and end-of-life care. *J Clin Oncol* 2007;25:715–23.

Quigley C. Opioid switching to improve pain relief and drug tolerability. *Cochrane Database Syst Rev* 2004, issue 3. CD004847. www.thecochranelibrary.com

Rubin SC, ed. *Chemotherapy of Gynecologic Cancers*, 2nd edn. Philadelphia: Lippincott Williams & Wilkins, 2004.

World Health Organization. *Cancer Pain Relief and Palliative Care. WHO Technical Report Series, 804.* Geneva: World Health Organization, 1990.

Future trends

Developments are likely in methods of screening and chemotherapy regimens. There is an increasing trend towards management tailored to the individual, with the general aim of minimizing toxicity while maximizing the chance of cure. Individualized treatments based on the genetic fingerprint of a patient may achieve both. Nanotechnology may open a new frontier for treatment. Diet and environment may unlock their secrets for the prevention and treatment of cancers.

Cervical neoplasia

Current screening programs are based on the original Papanicolaou methodology. However, great strides have been made in reducing laboratory errors. The computerized slide-review system continues to evolve as a useful means of double-checking results.

A therapeutic vaccine is certainly a near-term possibility and is now in clinical trials. Neoadjuvant chemotherapy may be directed by a predictive assay.

In the surgical arena, it seems likely that fertility-sparing procedures will become more widespread, particularly for women with small-volume tumors. For women with more advanced tumors, the combination of chemotherapy, radiotherapy and surgery may improve prognosis. Ultimately, reproductive organ cryopreservation and transplantation may eliminate cancer-associated infertility. Combination of treatment modalities including manipulation of light, oxygen and temperature may be introduced clinically. Proton therapy and other attempts to limit toxicity are fast becoming the standard of care.

Ovarian neoplasia

The most exciting potential for improving survival is in screening. Women with a family history of ovarian cancer are already routinely screened; it is to be hoped that this will become useful to all women in the not-too-distant future. Combinations of sophisticated laboratory and mathematical techniques may enable this. While genetic testing may have created many ethical dilemmas in the short term, such tests appear beneficial.

Chemotherapy regimens continue to improve, both in terms of efficacy and side effects. The relatively recent addition of targeted regimens has proved useful. Low-dose chemotherapy in combination with targeted therapy may be beneficial in women with advanced ovarian cancer, irrespective of surgical result. Refinement of intraperitoneal therapy may yield additional survival benefit.

Stem cells are being investigated as a cure and cause of cancers. Clinical trials of a related approach using dendritic cell vaccine have begun.

In 1977, the average survival following ovarian cancer was 10 months. By 2007, average survival exceeded 5 years. On average one new agent has become available every 5 years and, in the last 2–3 years, this has increased to seven to ten agents every year. This explosion in drug development coupled with new developments in genetic and tissue banking make the prospect of ovarian cancer becoming a chronic or curable disease all the more likely.

Vulvar neoplasia

Currently, vulvar neoplasia appears to present more commonly in younger women than in previously. This may be due to increasing levels of human papillomavirus and, possibly herpes simplex virus infection. The epidemiological trend is likely to stimulate basic research into the etiology of vulvar intraepithelial neoplasia progression. Surgical management is certainly moving towards more conservative surgery, and new methods of detecting lymph node involvement are being researched.

Uterine neoplasias

Radiation therapy has been refined to reduce toxicity. This may change the risk–benefit ratio to enhance its use in uterine cancer. Systemic treatment with chemotherapy and targeted therapies will find a useful place in the treatment of this disease.

In conclusion

While much remains to be done in the field of gynecologic oncology, the explosion in research over the last 20–30 years has reaped rich dividends for our patients. This is reflected in both increased survival times and an increasing cure rate. In addition, prevention rates for both cervical and endometrial cancer are increasing as a result of treatment of ascertained precursor lesions and vaccination. It is to be hoped that this trend continues.

Social and political advances may have the largest impact on cancer care. Reimbursement determines screening availability and access to new treatments. Socially determined disease related to obesity and the environment can affect an extremely large number of people. Patients and physicians must advocate for reform in healthcare delivery and increased research funding.

Useful resources

International

Cancer Council Australia
GPO Box 4708, Sydney NSW 2001
Level 1, 120 Chalmers St
Surry Hills NSW 2010
Tel: +61 2 8063 4100
info@cancer.org.au
www.cancer.org.au

National Centre for Gynaecological Cancer
Cancer Australia
PO Box 1201
Dickson ACT 2602
Tel: +61 2 6217 9818
gynaecentre@canceraustralia.gov.au
www.canceraustralia.gov.au/ncgc/
about-centre/ncgc-homepage

UK

Cancer Research UK
PO Box 123
Lincoln's Inn Fields
London WC2A 3PX
Tel: (Supporter Services) +44 (0)20
7121 6699
Tel: (Switchboard) +44 (0)20 7242
0200
www.cancerresearchuk.org

International Federation of Gynecology and Obstetrics
FIGO Secretariat, FIGO House,
Suite 3 – Waterloo Court
10 Theed Street
London, SE1 8ST
Tel: +44 20 7928 1166
www.FIGO.org

Jo's Trust (cervical cancer charity)
Tel: +44 (0)207 9367 498/7499
www.jotrust.co.uk

Macmillan Cancer Support
89 Albert Embankment
London SE1 7UQ
CancerLine: 0808 808 2020
Nurse info line: 0808 800
1234
www.macmillan.org.uk
www.cancerbackup.org.uk

Marie Curie Cancer Care
England
89 Albert Embankment
London SE1 7TP
Tel: +44 (0)20 7599 7777

Wales
Block C Mamhilad House
Mamhilad Park Estate
Pontypool
Torfaen NP4 0HZ
Tel: +44 (0)1495 740827
www.mariecurie.org.uk

USA
American Cancer Society
Tel: 1 800 ACS 2345 (or 1 866 228 4327)
www.cancer.org

American Congress of Obstetricians and Gynecologists
PO Box 96920
Washington, DC 20090–6920
Tel: +1 202 638 5577
resources@acog.org
www.acog.org

American Society for Colposcopy and Cervical Pathology
152 West Washington St
Hagerstown, MD 21740
Tel: +1 301 733 3640
Tel: 1 800 787 7227
www.asccp.org

Cancer*Care*
275 Seventh Ave, Floor 22
New York, NY 10001
Tel: 1 800 813 4673
info@cancercare.org
www.cancercare.org

National Comprehensive Cancer Network
275 Commerce Dr, Suite 300
Fort Washington, PA 19034
Tel: +1 215 690 0300
www.nccn.org

National Ovarian Cancer Coalition
2501 Oak Lawn Avenue
Suite 435
Dallas, Texas 75219
Tel: +1 214 273 4200
Helpline (US): 1-888-OVARIAN
nocc@ovarian.org

SHARE Self-help for women with breast or ovarian cancer
1501 Broadway
Suite 704A
New York, NY 10036
Tel: +1 212 719 0364
www.sharecancersupport.org

Further reading

Apgar BS, Brotzman GL, Spitzer M, eds. *Colposcopy Principles and Practice: An Integrated Textbook and Atlas.* Philadelphia: WB Saunders, 2002.

Berek JS, Hacker NF, eds. *Practical Gynecologic Oncology*, 4th edn. Philadelphia: Lippincott Williams & Wilkins, 2005.

Eifel PJ, Gershenson DM, Kavanagh JJ, Silva EG, eds. *Gynecologic Cancer.* MD Anderson Cancer Care Series. Texas: Springer Science, 2006.

Hoskins WJ, Perez CA, Young RC, Barakat RR, Markman M, Randall ME, eds. *Principles and Practice of Gynecologic Oncology*, 4th edn. Philadelphia: Lippincott Williams & Wilkins, 2005.

Kurman RJ, ed. *Blaustein's Pathology of the Female Genital Tract*, 5th edn. New York NY: Springer, 2002.

Smith JR, Del Priore G. *Women's Cancers: Pathways to Healing. A Patient's Guide to Dealing with Ovarian and Breast Cancer.* London: Springer, 2009.

Smith JR, Del Priore G, Cutin JP, Monaghan JM, eds. *An Atlas of Gynecologic Oncology: Investigation and Surgery*, 2nd edn. London: Taylor and Francis, 2005.

Smith JR, Healy J, Del Priore G, eds. *Atlas of Staging in Gynecological Cancer.* New York: Springer, 2008.

Index

141

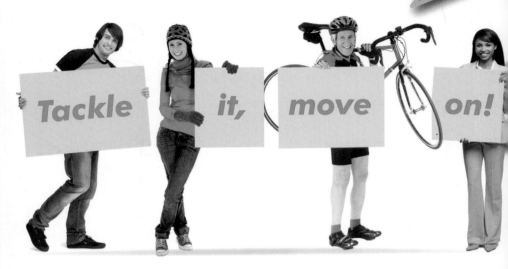